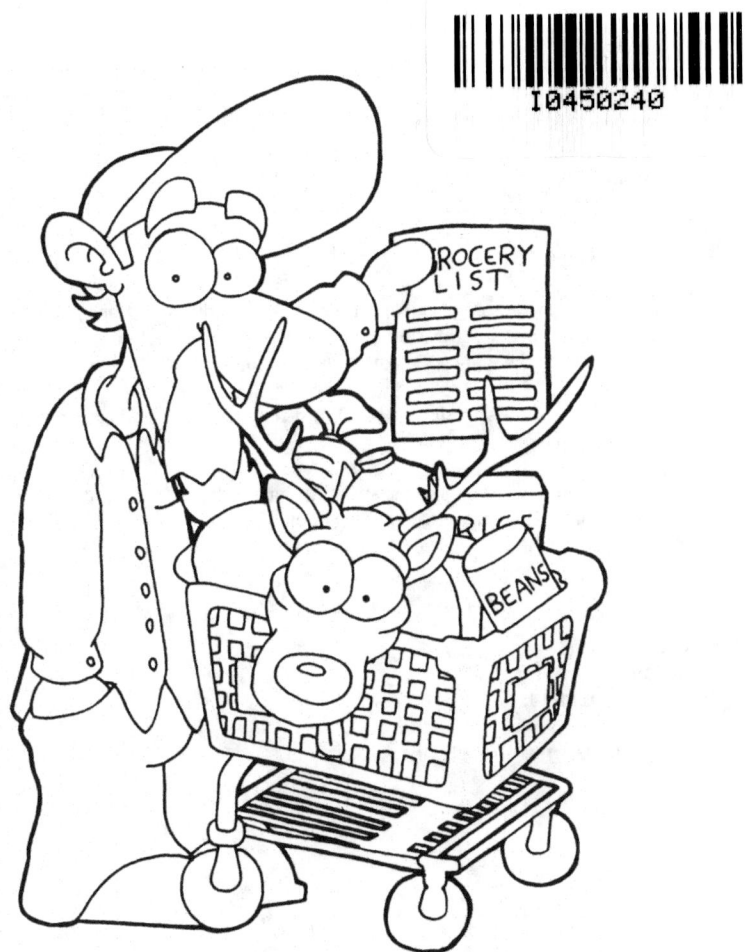

A Redneck's Guide
To Eatin' Right!

Written by Jeff Todd
(Ever heard of him? Probably not!)

Prologue

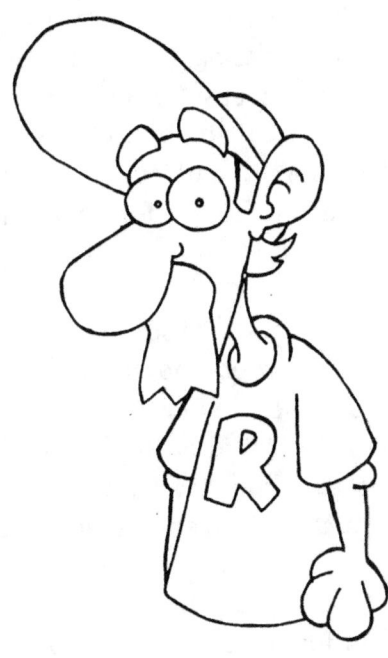

The book you're about to read is part of a ministry project that I have been working on for the past 7 years. It's not that I'm a slow writer or have bad typing skills. It's because it has been a growing faith journey.

Hi. My name is Jeff and I wrote this book. It is a result of my obedience to what the Lord has had me do. I basically used the gifts and talents that the Lord has given me to put this out there so that you can read. I'm nothing special and, to be honest, my English isn't that good either. But, it's a product of being faithful and true to something I feel that the Lord wanted me to do.

Who am I? I'm a simple man with a simple life and I live in a simple part of the world. Over the years, because of the current economic situation that has created a lot of problems in America, I have been sitting behind a laptop computer. I'm unemployed and this is what I've been doing with my time. This is my ministry.

Here's my testimony of how it came to be:

Before the economic meltdown, my wife and I ran a successful renovation business. As a company, we restored foreclosed homes for banks so that they could resell them in the market. We weren't wealthy by no means, but we made an honest living. There were times when business was extremely good and we were able to enjoy the finer things in life. The downfall was that we worked a lot, just like other people, chasing the American Dream. Sometimes it comes with a price. It's easy to put money as a number one priority in life. Because of our bad choice, I realize now that we were hurting our family and our self. We neglected our duties as parents and were to blame for some of the problems that our kids were having at the time.

The wake-up call came to us when my son got into some serious trouble in school. He was at the end of his rope and was placed in a holding cell for something he had done. He was scared and needed someone to turn to. This was the day that he accepted Jesus as his Lord and Savior. It was also the day that we, as parents, realized our life was in a mess. We were saved, but hadn't been living like it.

At that moment, my wife and I prayed for the Lord to take over. We gave Him our life, our business, and our family and said, "You can have it all. Use us for Your glory." And Jesus rescued us that day.

You would think that He would take a prayer like that and simply take the life we had and move forward. But, no. Our life from that point seemed to go downhill. Over time, we lost our business, our money, and our selfish pride. But, at the same time, He provided our needs and even paid off our car and our home. We were jobless, yet we were taken care of. Instead of having the finer things in life, we had what we needed – no more, no less.

In the midst of the chaos, this ministry started. It was during a time when social networking websites were popular (MySpace, Facebook, etc). I felt the calling to write and post them on these sites for people to read. They were called blogs and it was a popular thing to do. Social networking was the latest fad and millions of people were doing it. It was a great way to share Jesus with people.

I felt my purpose was to teach from the Bible and share my life's experiences that would relate to scriptures from the Bible. It seemed every day I learned something new and I had to write it down. It was sorta like from the movie Forrest Gump when he was asked why he ran across America. He simply said, "Cause I felt like running."

It was like this for me. I felt like writing and it went on for a few years. Over time, I had accumulated a lot of stuff.

I received some advice from a friend. He told me that I should start creating books. Technology had came a long way and self-publishing a book was free and easy to use. So, I went that route. This is a part of what you hold in your hand right now.

Thank you for taking the time to read this. I hope it is a blessing to you.

Introduction

Every creature that walks, crawls, swims, flies or slithers on this planet has one thing in common. Yep! That's right! We all have stomachs.

A stomach is that organ-thing in our bodies that looks kinda like a bag. Am I right? It's purpose is to hold all of that food we put into it and share it – all of the nutrients, vitamins and all the other crap – to our many body parts to help us survive. And because we have stomachs, that means we all have to eat. It's how the whole ecosystem thing works. We eat, we live and we poop. That's pretty much it in a nutshell. You with me?

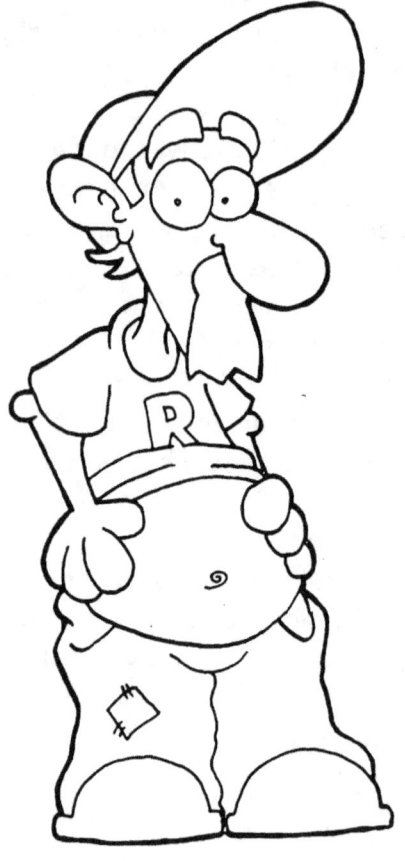

In case you didn't know, all creatures on this planet depend on each other for survival. This is called the 'food chain'. Humans are at the top of the chain and we eat animals that eat other animals that eat other animals and this continues until there is nothing left to eat. It keeps the environment clean, healthy and nothing is wasted. It's a perfect system – a rotating cycle that keeps everything flowing in a positive direction. Right?

But, if you look at the world around you, there are a lot of people with health issues and most doctors blame it on poor diets, lack of exercise and unhealthy eating habits. They should know because they are skilled, trained and certified at what they do. They have put years and thousands of 'educational dollars' into studying the human body to know what it takes to make it work and what doesn't.

Now, I'm no genius or a certified dietary consultant, but I do see a lot of unhealthy people barely able to walk around in the world today and I believe their eating habits has a lot to do with it. Somewhere along the line, we've changed the flow of how things were originally meant to be.

There's another factor that plays in all of this - some people are just flat out lazy. We tend to sit around for most of the day

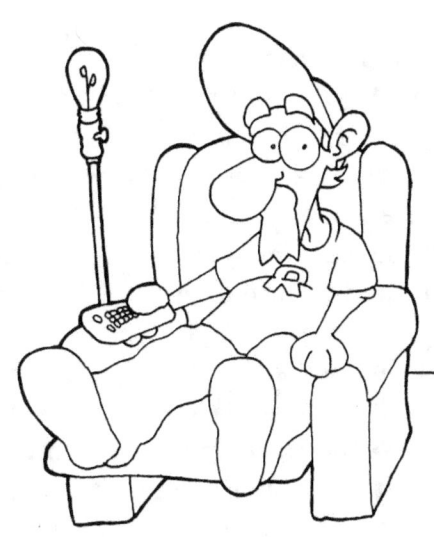

entertaining ourselves with the most up-to-date techno-devices and it seems everything is handed to us. The only exercise we may get is from the use of our thumbs and occasionally walking to the bathroom. Life has become easier than it used to be before all of these modern conveniences became part of our every day world. It's not good for the body, but its just how it is.

Don't get me wrong. I love the

fact that I can change the channel on my TV by simply pressing a button on a remote control while sitting in my recliner. I think it's awesome that I no longer have to hunt for my own food or make my own clothes. That's why we have Wally World right down the road. I can buy everything I need and these conveniences are there at my fingertips. That's cool! But, there's not a whole lot of physical activity that goes into it on my part to get what I want.

Take a look at most of the kids out there. Many of them are fat and lazy. Back in my day when I was a kid, we would go outside and play. This was good exercise. It was good for the body and we loved it. When was the last time you saw a kid playing in the yard? Kids these days barely get out of their rooms. They sit with their little game controllers in their hands, ear plugs in their ears and a bag of chips and a sugary drink off to the side somewhere putting water stains on our furniture. Something isn't right about this picture. This 'easy life' has created some unhealthy children and parents have became too busy with every day activities to correct them. Folks, it's only going to get worse.

Obesity isn't the only problem we're facing in society today. There are a bunch of skinny people out there that don't eat properly either. They think eating a leaf or two is healthy as long as they chase it down with water. No! Many of them think that they have to follow the media trends of 'being skinny' to be popular. No! Looking anorexic is not something you want to be. It's a medical condition that needs medical attention.

It's a messed up world that we live in and I am part of it, too. I'm just as guilty as anyone else out there because I know I don't eat all of the right foods or exercise like I should. I mean, right now I am sitting here typing on a laptop when I should be upstairs in the kitchen fixing me something to eat for lunch. But, no! I'll still be here typing until I start feeling dizzy from starving myself all day. I'm no different than anyone else.

My daily routine usually consists of 2 glasses of black coffee for breakfast in the morning. I don't use sugar or cream because it makes my coffee taste like pancake syrup. This is my breakfast and coffee has no real health benefit. If anything, since coffee is considered a diuretic, it flushes out any possible nutrients that I may have.

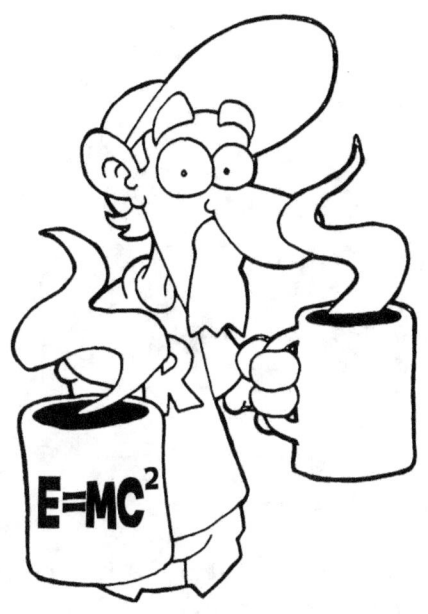

When lunch rolls around, I eat three potted meat sandwiches because they're convenient and they taste good. Most people don't eat potted meat sandwiches because of the stuff that goes into its ingredients. Hog guts and intestines may not look too appealing to some people out there.

Dinner time is different. I eat a huge plate full of whatever my wife decides to cook. Dinner around my house is usually a quick meal straight out of a box because nobody has the time or energy to cook something healthy. We eat it because, if anyone complains about what's for dinner, they get fussed at and told to go make a sandwich. Nobody wants a sandwich for dinner. It's more of a lunch food.

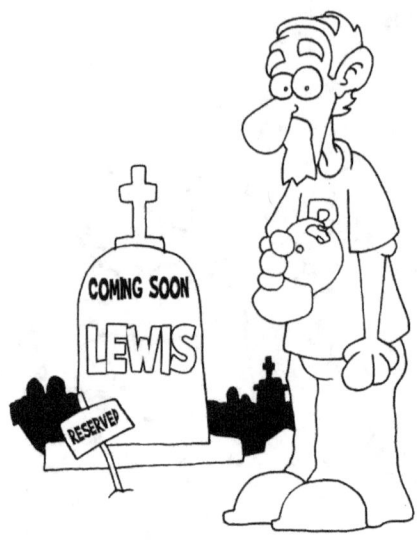

Was my day full of healthy choices? Definitely, no! Hey! I'm just like most folks out there. But, if we're going to change this vicious cycle that we're in, we're going to have to take the time to look deeper into what we're putting into our bodies and what we should be doing to keep our bodies healthier. Our current lifestyle is pushing us closer to an early grave... and FAST.

As with most problems in life, the first step towards change is to first know that there is a problem. We have to wake up and make some changes. If you can't see your feet when you stand up, there's a problem. If you get out of breath by simply walking up steps, there's a problem. If your doctor has warned you time and time again to change your diet and get plenty of exercise, it's because there's a reason... you have a problem!

What's the solution? We can go to the bookstore and stock up on all of the 'How To' books for advice, but everyone has their own

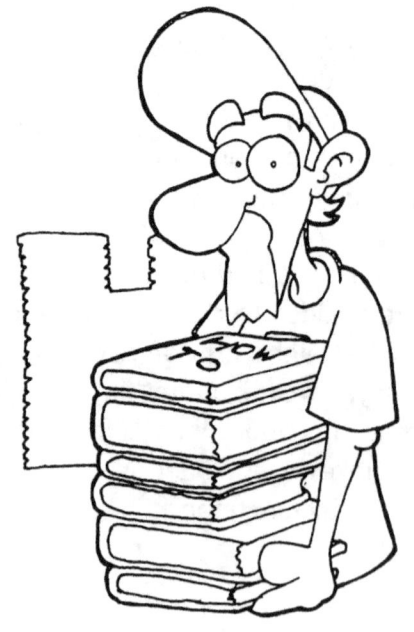

opinion. Some don't work. We could visit a health consultant or a nutritionist. They're pretty smart on this type of thing, but it could cost you a fortune. Or, we could sign up for the latest diet or exercise craze. It may work for a couple of months and then we get bored with it and go back to where we started.

For me, the Bible is the source for all information. It is God's words to us to help us live better. Just like most problems we face in the world today, we can turn to the Bible to provide us with the solutions on how to fix it. That's what it's there for.

That's the purpose of this guide today. As I learn from the Bible

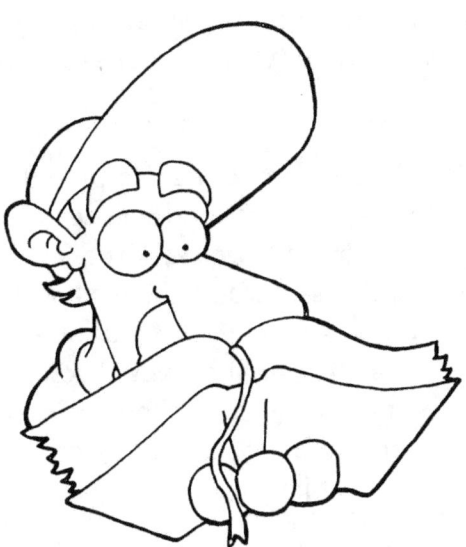

what it says to me about how and what to eat, I'll gladly share it with you. No problem! We can learn together and make the proper changes in our life that is required to help us live healthier, happier and live longer. That's part of God's perfect plan for us and it's in the Bible. All we have to do is read it and apply it. You agree?

What's The Problem?

And God said, Behold, I have given you every herb bearing seed, which is upon the face of all the earth, and every tree, in the which is the fruit of a tree yielding seed; to you it shall be for meat. - Genesis 1: 29

And God blessed Noah and his sons, and said unto them, Be fruitful, and multiply, and replenish the earth. And the fear of you and the dread of you shall be upon every beast of the earth, and upon every fowl of the air, upon all that moveth upon the earth, and upon all the fishes of the sea; into your hand are they delivered. Every moving thing that liveth shall be meat for you; even as the green herb have I given you all things. - Genesis 9: 1-3

From the very beginning of time, God created life. He provided man and woman with a wide assortment of food choices. But because of sin, they had to leave paradise to go work the land — by creating their own gardens, planting seeds and doing all of the stuff required to put food on the table. If they wanted a

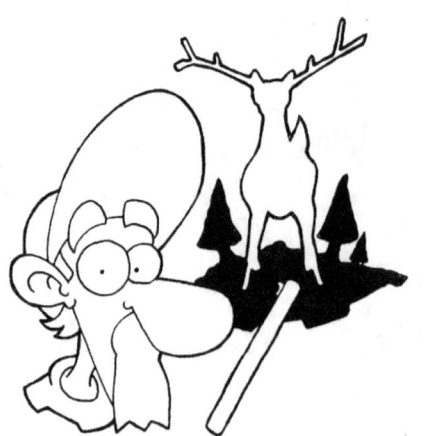

hamburger, they would actually have to go out there, kill the cow and process it. McDonald's wasn't invented yet.

This took a lot of work and exercise on their part to provide a meal for the day. And since refrigerators weren't created yet, every day was an attempt to get food. You couldn't sleep in and order take-out later. If they wanted breakfast, they had to get up early enough to go get it. The same would apply for lunch and dinner. It took an effort.

The great thing about all of this was that all of their food was fresh. It wasn't imported from China or from a huge factory that packed the food with preservatives and artificial junk. It didn't get touched by everybody's hands on an assembly line somewhere. This stuff came straight out of the ground, off of a tree and from their own backyard. They knew where it came from and didn't need to question it.

Over time, I'm sure things began evolving. People got smarter and created new innovative ways of doing things. These so-called improvements were made to get us to where we are today. If I had to sum it all up from creation to now, I imagine it went down a little something like this:

Years passed since Day 1. Food was great, but the labor involved in getting it was rough. Man's hands were tough with callouses. They complained about sore backs and achy muscles. Everybody's neck had become 'red' from all of the sun they received from working the fields all day.

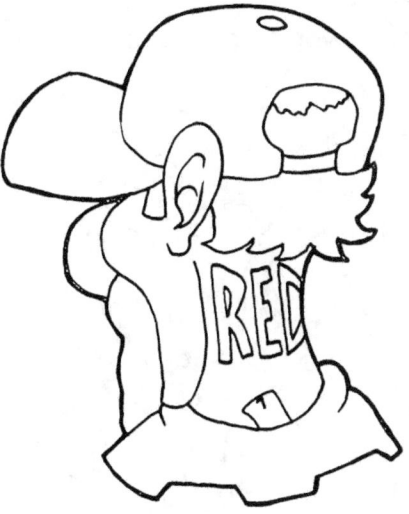

Note: The term 'redneck' may have originated during this time.

It wasn't too long afterward that money was created. Also, at the same time, salesmen arose from the dusty fields. These salesmen came up with a brilliant idea and plan that man would no longer have to work the field for food anymore. They could actually do other things and earn money instead. They could exchange this hard-earned money for food that they could purchase directly from the salesmen. It sounded like a great idea for the both of them.

Food was now being mass produced in high quantities, as a business, by the salesmen, and could be sold. Man liked this idea because it meant he no longer had to get blisters on his hands or be sore from muscle aches from all that exercise in the field. They could now focus on other important things on their To-Do lists or doing leisure activities such as playing golf or going to rock concerts with their buddies. The downside of all of this would be that they had to depend on these salesmen to provide their food and trust them that the food they were supplying was safe for human consumption. But, at least they didn't have to work the land anymore. That was some very hard work! Now their world was advancing and they liked where it was heading.

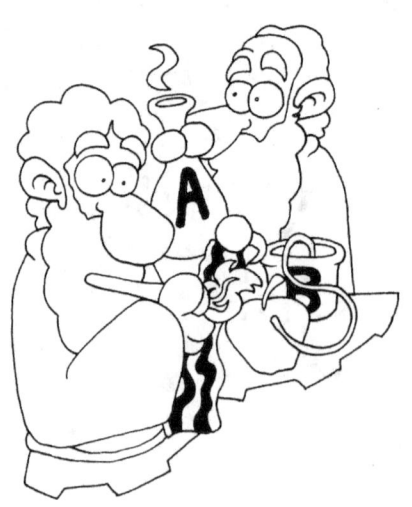

As the population began to grow, the demand for food from these salesmen increased. The land was getting overpopulated, people were forced to move outward and salesmen had to create new innovative ways to distribute food to their customers that lived far away. The problem was that their fresh food wouldn't be fresh by the time it got to them. I would guess that, by this time, scientists were invented.

I can see a group of folks, now called scientists, sitting around, thinking and coming up with ways to preserve food. They may have tried a few experiments to see if their latest concoction worked for the common folk. Maybe they sprinkled a little of this and that on some Grade A Choice meat and shipped it to their customers. If the customers ate it and they didn't die or get sick, it was a keeper. If they died, well, they knew not to try that again.

As the population continued to grow, the demand for food kept increasing. These salesmen were busy and had to pick up the pace in productivity. They needed to produce more food and do it rather quickly. So, they had a meeting with the scientists. Together they came up with a brilliant plan.

"Let's inject all of our food with Concoction XYZ because it makes it grow bigger, faster and almost tastes the same. Plus, after a few more years, the general public won't even know the difference anyway."

So they did.

This worked wonderfully. Money was good for the salesmen. Then, greed stepped in and the salesmen wanted to make more profits for their goods. They heard a rumor that a country nearby was working at lower hourly rates. They could supply what the salesmen were already getting from their current workers at a fraction of the cost. Yeah, the salesmen may not know exactly how these foreigners produced their food or what they put in it, but as long as the finished product looked the same, they could sell it. This is when the importing and exporting business began and business was very good.

During the same time, the world began modernizing. Cool gadgets were being invented to make life easier. Man no longer had to walk to find entertainment. They could now be entertained from the convenience of their own homes. Even in the work place, machines were built to replace the hard labor that was once supplied from the workers. Most of these workers got assigned desk jobs and spent more time pressing buttons to keep the machines going. It was work, but mostly mental labor. The physical side of labor slowly began to decrease while every one's waistline began to expand. But, this wasn't a problem because the latest trend at that time was that 'being fat was cool'.

Many years passed and health problems became a growing concern around the world. People were getting sick, dying younger and no one could figure out why. Yeah, this created another new business. People were becoming doctors, this new thing called 'medicine' was invented, hospitals were being built and the demand for these services was booming. Business was good.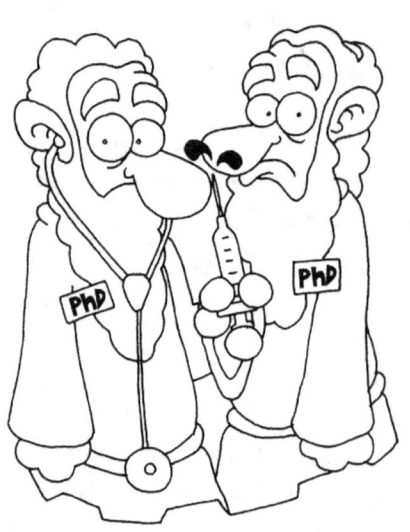

Basically, over the course of time, healthy people became unhealthy and lazy, while businesses in the food and medical industry flourished.

I know this whole story sounds a little farfetched. But, there is some truth in it. This brings us to the world we live in today. Sound familiar?

It all narrows down to two basic problems:

People don't eat right
People don't exercise

Let's face it. We really don't know what we are eating today. We buy food based on how pretty the box is on the shelf or how awesome media makes it look on commercials and advertisements. We don't read the ingredients or learn about where it originally comes from or how it was processed. And when we eat it, we don't exercise or move around to work all of this junk off. The next thing we know, we have accumulated a lot of medical debt because now we are unhealthy.

Life, from the very beginning, was about working the land and eating the fruit of our labor. It was an even balance of eating and exercise. Both worked together hand in hand. Can we honestly say we are doing that today? No. We have a problem.

Food
Is It A Problem?

"You are what you eat."

I'm sure you've heard that saying before. It's not a Bible verse, but there's a lot of truth in it. Before I explain, let's think on these questions:

What foods do we currently eat?
Where does our food come from?
What's actually in it?

Most of what we eat comes from a grocery store somewhere. It would be great if we had the time to grow a garden and hunt for our own food like the people did from the old days. But, the reality is that we don't have time in our daily schedule to do it. We rely on others to do it for us. We have gotten so busy that it's easier to just pay them for it. Am I right?

My wife and I have tried to grow gardens before. It's a lot of hard work and when you compare your results with what you can get from the grocery store, it seems its better to just buy our own fruits and vegetables. I mean, there's a lot involved in growing a garden.

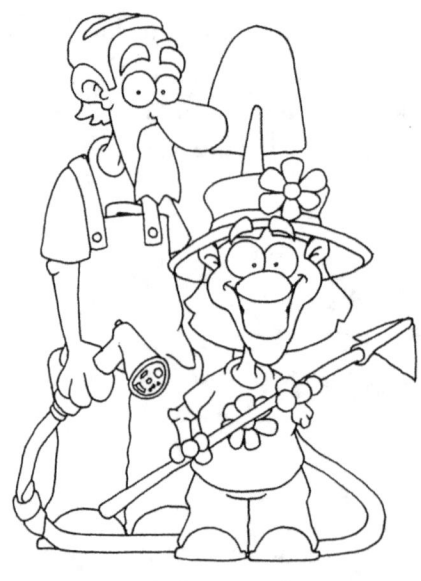

A few years ago was a good example. My wife and I were excited to get our garden started. We picked a nice spot in our yard that would receive a good bit of sunshine. We knew that in order to have a great garden, it would require sunlight. We dug up the ground to loosen the soil. We tried this at first by hand by using a shovel, but it made us so sore that we decided to rent a plow instead from a our local equipment rental store. Yeah, it cost us about $100, but to us it was well worth it.

We wanted to make a big garden with beans, cucumbers, okra, squash, watermelon, corn and several other types of vegetables and fruit. We were serious about it. We made rows from the softened soil. We planted seeds within the rows every few inches apart just like the instructions on the seed pack told us to do. We added some fertilizer and gave it its first dose of fresh water from the garden hose. It was beautiful. We were so proud, but definitely tired.

We made it a daily routine to water the ground. We knew the importance of fresh water and how it would help the garden grow because we read about it in one of those gardening magazines. After a few weeks, we started seeing those seeds we planted begin to sprout. Little green plants started popping out of the ground all over the place. They were growing everywhere, including places that we know we didn't even plant a seed. It was so cool! We later learned 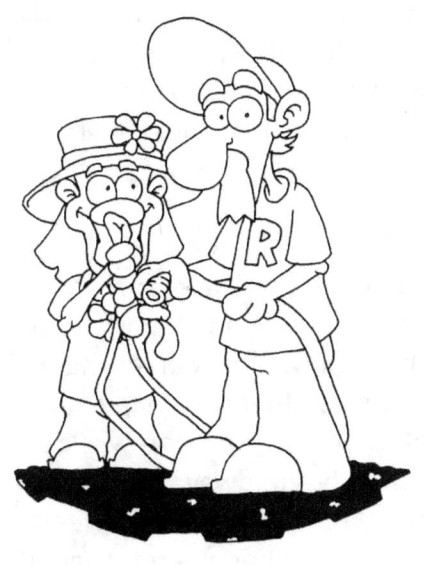 that these were the bad plants called 'weeds' and they grew much faster than the good plants. So, we spent the next couple of months every day trying to keep them pulled out. This was hard work.

Everything seemed to be going great. The new plants started budding with beautiful flowers in various colors. The flowers started turning into small vegetables and fruit. This was a major accomplishment for us that we couldn't wait to share the news with our children. We thought, "Years from now, we can tell our grandchildren about our successful garden just like our grandparents used to tell us. Wouldn't that be awesome? They will think we are like superheroes with pitchforks and garden rakes."

The vegetables were finally ready to pick. We filled a basket full of squash and cucumbers and we proudly carried them home and put them on the kitchen counter. Yes, they were small as compared to the ones we could buy from the grocery store. But, it didn't matter. These were ours – we grew these. We knew they would taste much better than anything we could ever buy anywhere else. These were fresh. We watched them grow and knew exactly what was in them.

Unfortunately, some of the vegetables didn't do so well. We had a hot and dry Summer that year. Many of the tomatoes shriveled up to nothing and died. The corn grew tall and was beginning to show a few ears, but a sudden wind knocked most of them down and killed them. We may have gotten about ten ears of corn out of it. The watermelon was doing good until it decided to split in half about midway to being ripe. The bugs ate up our cauliflower and broccoli. And one weekend, we decided to take a quick vacation. When we returned, it looked like a big fat elephant sat right down in the middle of our garden and killed everything its butt landed on. It broke our hearts because we didn't know what we did wrong. Everything we worked so hard for just died in a matter of days and we weren't there to help.

We ended up getting about an eighth of what we planted. Was it worth the money and effort? Probably not. That could be why many people go to the grocery store instead. It's seems to be more practical and it saves you money in the long run. Is it the best way? I don't know.

We have to place a lot of trust in our grocery stores the companies that produce the food and our government to make sure that the foods we are buying are safe. I'm sure that food products, just like most of the stuff in stores today, are probably being outsourced to some foreign land. We can only hope that they are following all of the same guidelines that are required by the FDA (Food & Drug Administration). We assume, that if the grocery store has it on their shelves, it's ready and healthy for us to eat. Right?

And because of economic reasons, we also buy food based on what we can afford. If we are barely making ends meet, we will buy foods that are cheap, on sale or the ones that we have coupons for. To create meals for a week, we have to stretch our hard-earned dollars to get enough food to feed us until we get paid again. That's basic economics.

On the flipside, if a company wants to sell their 'food product', they have to create it so that it is affordable, even if it means creating shortcuts or adding foods with filler to make it look like we're getting a good deal for our money. Because of this, financially deprived people like myself tend to buy and eat foods

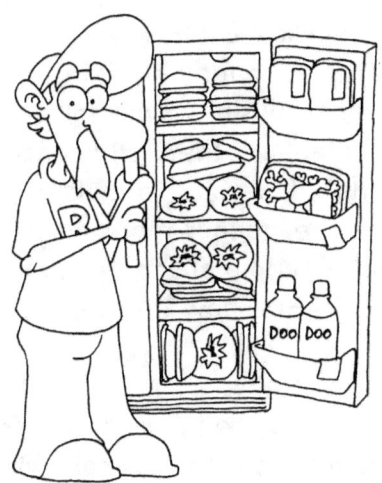

that are probably not good for us. But that's all we can afford, so we buy it.

In my home, like most people, our refrigerator is stocked with chicken and hamburger meat. The main reasons are because they're cheap and there's a hundred different ways to cook and eat them. You can mix them with other ingredients from a box and have a different meal every night. You know what I'm saying?

Is chicken or hamburger meat bad for us? I guess that depends on how we cook it and where it originally comes from. We all know that the food we buy more than likely comes from a grocery store. We should look deeper into it than that by going beyond the grocery store shelf and towards the original source.

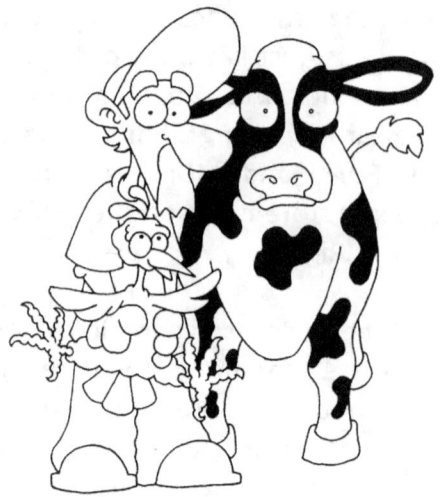

Where did these animals come from that offer the meat that stores put on their shelves? Did they come from a farm? If so, what kind of farm and what were these animals fed while they lived there? How were their living conditions? Was the environment nasty? If 'we are what we eat', then we become whatever these animals had as part of their diets, too.

The Food Industry is a business. And just like most businesses out there, the key is to produce more goods and offer it at affordable prices. The problem is in what steps a business will take to produce more and become more profitable. If they sell beef by the pound, some may pump a cow full of steroids to make the animal bigger. Since meat is sold by the pound, more weight equals more profits. Yeah, there will be people out there eating contaminated food filled with chemicals. But, hey! It's business! Right?

If a company sells green beans in a can, they could use fertilizer that makes a garden grow overnight. Yeah, their customers will be eating a bunch of weird chemicals, but at least the company is producing products at a super fast pace to meet the demands. Or maybe they could shoot some preservatives in it so that it would last forever. No waste equals more profits, too. So what if it rots your stomach out and makes you pee blood. It's business! And its profitable!

It's a good idea to know what we are putting in our bodies. Beef isn't just cow meat anymore. Oh no! There are other hands involved in putting that chunk of ground round on the shelves at the grocery store. There could be stuff in it that could be harmful to our bodies. It's best to do our homework.

Personal Case Study #1
Checking Out The Ingredients

As I got deeper into this whole writing project, I decided to take a look at we eat as a family in my home. I wanted to know what we were actually putting into our bodies. This is my personal case study.

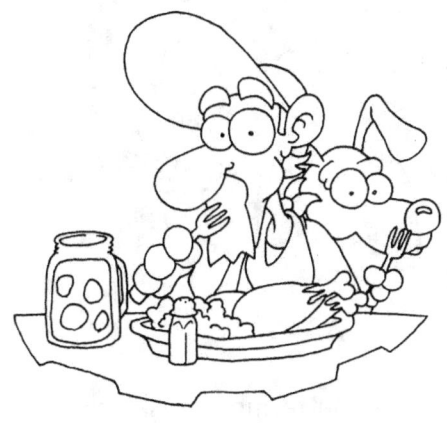

Dinner at our house is pretty simple. We will pull a pack of meat from the freezer and let it thaw out throughout the day. When it's time to cook, we'll grab a few cans of vegetables (corn and some kind of bean) from the pantry, maybe a box of macaroni and cheese and sometimes we'll top it all off with some dinner rolls that were already cooked somewhere else. All we have to do is heat it up. That's a dinner for us on any given night. It's plain and simple. For rednecks like me, this is eating in-style at the highest level. As my wife would say, the alternative would be "if you don't like what I cooked, go fix yourself a sandwich." So, we learned to eat what she cooks.

Here's a closer look at tonight's meal:

Cubed steak (pre-packaged)
Whole Kernel Corn (from a can)
Sweet Peas (from a can)
Macaroni & Cheese (from a box)
No bread tonight (ran out of dinner rolls)

Cubed Steak

This was purchased from the grocery store and looks harmless. It's pink and pre-chopped for easy eating. I'm sure it came from a cow somewhere – possibly in the United States. We're really not sure. There's not much to know about the poor cow that this meat came from. I couldn't tell you what his eating habits were or if he got a great bill of health from his local doctor. All I know is that it wouldn't be in the grocery store if it wasn't 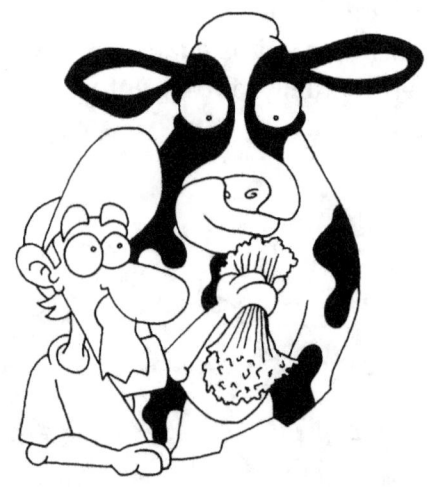 safe to eat. I also know that we will be battering it up in flour and frying it in a pan.

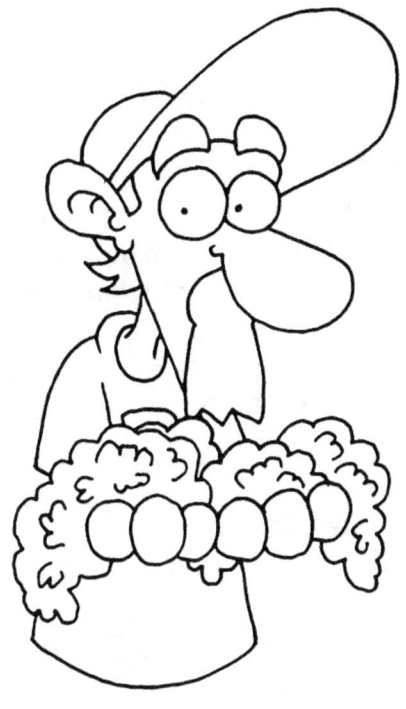

Is there a health concern? There is when I am forced to think about it. They say 'fried foods' is bad for you. Plus, there are articles all over the Internet that talk about additives that are mixed in with ground beef to make it look like you're getting more meat for your hard-earned dollar. Their way of thinking is that "as long as its pink, regardless of what you mix with it, it's considered meat". People don't question 'pink' meat sold in the grocery store. If it were blue or had traces of green chunks in it, people would get all crazy and that store would be on the 6 o'clock news. Pink is good. Right?

I also learned that ground beef is chemically treated with ammonia to kill bacteria. Ammonia? Really? Yep! Not only can you clean your toilet with it, your food gets cleaned with it, too. And we're eating it. Sounds yummy, huh?

Ever wonder how many hands touched your food before you? I'm sure it's not something you would want to think about. But, food gets handled just like any other product out there that's being manufactured. It seems every business has some kind of assembly line with conveyor belts and fast product-moving machinery. I'm sure there are some in the food business, too. These workers probably don't see this as food anymore, but more like a product. They touch it, breathe on it, sneeze on it and whatever else. But, hey! At least they squirt it down with ammonia to kill all that nasty bacteria off! Kinda gross, huh?

Whole Kernel Corn (from a can)

This is a can of corn that's really no different than anything else you would buy from the grocery store. Ours is not a 'name brand' item because we try to save money whenever we can. I'm sure it will taste the same. The ingredients tell me that it is made from corn, water, sugar and salt. All of these ingredients sound familiar and that would make it healthy. It's made from all natural ingredients. Right?

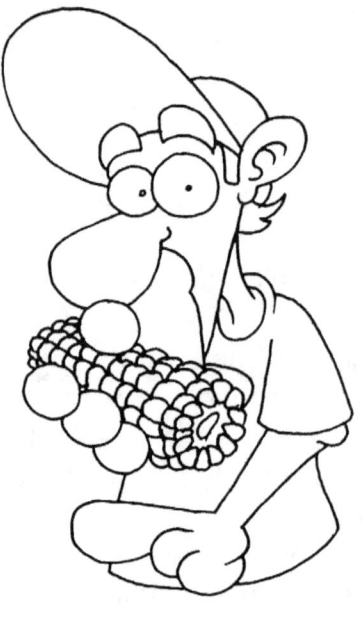

Is there a health concern? At first glance, probably not. But, then again, we don't really know who grew this stuff. We don't know the whole farming history. What if they used harmful pesticides and fertilizers? What if bugs fell inside the big corn mixing bowl? We wouldn't know about it. They don't put stuff like that on the product label. FDA doesn't require it as long they meet the standard bug allowance numbers, so why should they try and scare customers off?

I did notice, however, that this corn does contain a bunch of salt. I assume the salt in the ingredients is used as a preservative and is considered harmless. But from what I've read, large amounts of salt could lead to high blood pressure. But, who ever considers that kind of stuff anyway? Salt is salt and the number on the Nutrition Facts doesn't really make any sense.

Sweet Peas (from a can)

Here's another great canned item. This time it's sweet peas that came directly from aisle 5 at our local grocery store. The ingredients tell me that it contains sweet peas, water, sugar and salt.

Sounds naturally safe, doesn't it? Actually studies show that peas in their natural form are good for you. I've read where peas were low in fat and high in protein, fiber, vitamins and nutrients. Some studies say that peas prevent stomach cancer, wrinkles and help regulate blood sugar. So, peas have to be good for you. The only potential problem I see in eating this is the high amounts of sodium and not knowing the 'farming' story. It would be the same risks as the canned corn that we mentioned earlier.

One thing I noticed from my farming experience is that these sweet peas aren't the same color 'green' as the peas I grew in my garden a few years back. Maybe this is what 'real' peas should look like. Mine may have gotten too much sun? Who knows?

Macaroni & Cheese (from a box)

This is my kids' favorite side dish. It is their first choice any time we go out to eat. It appears to be an innocent food. I mean, all it has in it is noodles with powdery cheese poured on it, right? Let's read the ingredients on the side of the box:

- Enriched macaroni product (wheat flour, niacin, iron [ferrous sulfate], thiamine mononitrate, riboflavin, folic acid)
- Cheddar cheese sauce (cheddar cheese [milk, cheese

27

culture, salt, enzymes], water, whey, canola oil, sodium phosphate, whey protein concentrate, nonfat milk, salt, contains 2% or less of the following: sodium alginate, lactic acid, preservative [sorbic acid], color [oleoresin paprika, apocarotenal]

That's a lot of ingredients with a bunch of big words on the label. Most of these words I haven't even heard or seen before. I don't want to question it because I don't want people thinking I'm dumb. Is this a healthy food?

I don't know, but based on what I've read, there are a lot of additives in this stuff to make me not want to eat it. I

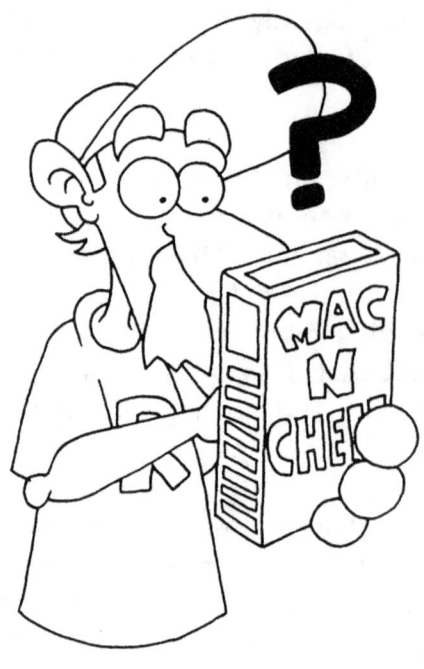

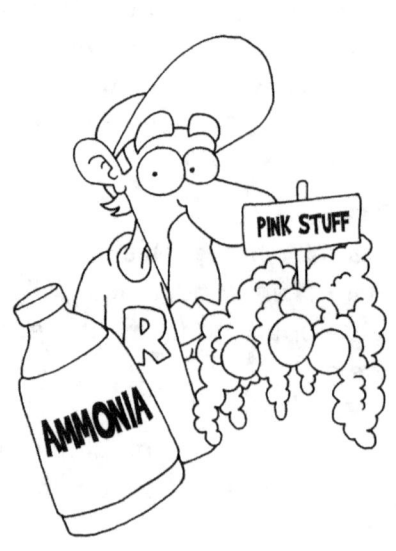

read somewhere that sodium phosphate is linked to kidney damage. That's pretty scary to know.

Basically, what I have learned from doing a personal case study on tonight's meal is that I am eating ammonia and some kind of 'unknown' pink stuff. I could also be risking the chances of getting high blood pressure and kidney damage from eating a simple dinner like this. I wonder how many other meals we've eaten that could have been a risk to our lives, too. I don't know!

When was the last time you read the ingredients on your food? You might find some disturbing information after ding a little bit of research. It could change the way you eat.

Nutritional Facts
It's Best To Know The Facts

There's another tidbit of information placed on most foods we buy at the grocery store. It's called Nutrition Facts. We've all seen it printed on the packaging, but probably never put much thought into it. For many of us, these words and numbers don't make a whole lot of sense. But they are important.

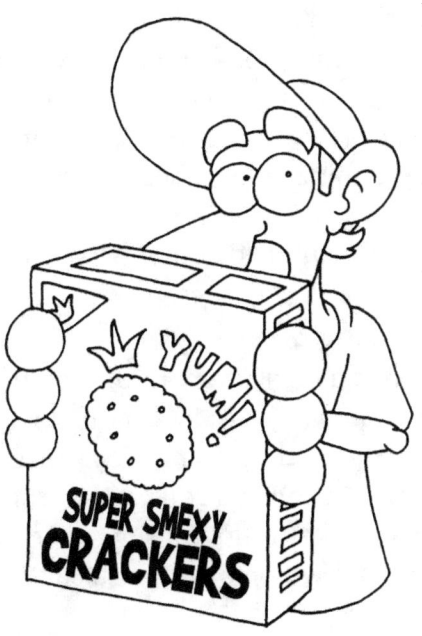

I think for the most part, people eat foods based on how pretty the picture looks on the outside of the box. I know I do. It starts with a craving inside our brains. We walk to the kitchen and begin looking around for pictures of food that we think will satisfy us. I guess that's why junk food appeals to our brain so easily. It's the picture on its packaging that lures us in.

Most junk food packaging has pictures of happy people eating happy food. Everybody is smiling. Some food items have cool cartoon characters on it that make it appealing to kids or parents that are in-tune with their 'inner child'. All of this creative marketing makes junk food our first choice when we are looking for something to eat. Right?

The fact is, our bodies are craving nutrition. It is looking for nutrients – vitamins, proteins and other body essentials. This is why we should learn to ignore all of the pretty pictures on food labels and focus on what is really important.

Nutrition Facts is one of the most important parts of the food label. By reading it, you can find out how much fat, protein and fiber the food has in it. It's a breakdown of all of the nutritional stuff that's in the food that is prepared by the food company's nutritional department. It is regulated by law and the format looks the same way for any food we buy. When we learn how to read it, we can compare it with other food choices and determine what is best for us.

Here's a breakdown of what is contained in the Nutrition Facts:

Serving Size
This is a measurement of food that reflects how much an average person will eat in one helping. Serving size is explained in 'kitchen' terms using words like cups, spoons, slices and also in grams. Serving size is set by the FDA, not by the food company that makes it, for all similar products so that you can compare it without whipping out a calculator.

The actual serving size may vary per family. In my home we

generally multiply it by 2. I'm sure its not healthy, but we like to eat.

Servings Per Package
The next line tells you how many servings the package will have in it. This will help you compare similar products on the basis of costs per serving. Multiply this number by the serving size and it should equal, or come pretty close to, the total volume of the package.

This section is also good for determining how many boxes or cans of this food you will need for the amount of people you plan to feed. In my case, I have to feed 8 people that eat double servings. Yeah, that's a lot of math and a lot of food.

Calories
This line tells you the number of calories per serving.

Calories From Fat
This line tells you how many calories in each serving are from fat.

Percent Daily Value (DV)
This section tells you what percentage of the total recommended daily amount of each nutrient (fats, carbohydrates, proteins, major vitamins, and minerals) is in each serving, based on a 2,000 calorie per day diet. These values cannot be applied to babies or kids under four.

Each person's calorie intake could be different. Consult someone certified in this area of expertise that knows all about calories. Do the math to figure out what is right for you and your family.

Total Fat

This line tells you how many grams of fat is in one serving and what percent this is of the recommended daily value (DV). For example, *Total Fat 1 gram, 2%* means that one serving would contain one gram of fat and two percent of the total recommended daily intake of fat. Even the factory fats (hydrogenated and partially hydrogenated) must legally be listed in the total fat.

Saturated Fat

This subheading under *Total Fat* tells you how much of the fat in each serving is saturated fat and what percent this is of your daily recommended value (DV).

Cholesterol

This line tells you how many milligrams of cholesterol and what percent this is of the recommended daily value.

Sodium

This line refers to salt. The DV for sodium is less than 2,400 mg a day.

Potassium

The recommended DV for potassium is 3,500 mg a day.

Total Carbohydrates

Dietary fiber
Sugars
Other carbohydrates

Total carbohydrate: This tells you how many grams of carbohydrates are in each serving and the percentage of the Daily Value this represents. This number includes starches, complex carbohydrates, dietary fiber, added sugar sweeteners, and non-digestible additives. The following three carbohydrates all add up to the total carbohydrate value.

Dietary fiber: This figure represents the number of grams of fiber in each serving.

Sugars: This figure represents the number of grams of added sweeteners, which may appear in the ingredients list as: sugar, corn syrup, honey, brown sugar, etc.

Other carbohydrates: This line reveals the number of grams of complex carbohydrates, not including fiber, but including non-digestible additives, such as stabilizers and thickening agents.

Protein
This line tells you how many grams of protein are in each serving. You will notice that the percent DV is missing from the protein label because protein insufficiency is not usually thought to be a problem.

Vitamins and Minerals
This list includes the percentage of the recommended daily allowance for vitamins A and C, calcium and iron in each serving. The food may provide significant amounts of other vitamins and minerals, which may also be listed, though not required by law.

Ingredients
The ingredients list tells you, usually in fine print, what ingredients the food contains. These are listed in order, starting with the ingredient found in the largest amount, by weight and progressing to the ingredient present in the smallest amount. I actually first learned about this from my wife several years ago.

The ingredients list may be the most important information on the box to someone with food allergies or to a parent who is concerned about the effects of food coloring or preservatives on their child's behavior. Here you can find out if a food contains eggs, soy, milk, corn or whatever you must avoid eating.

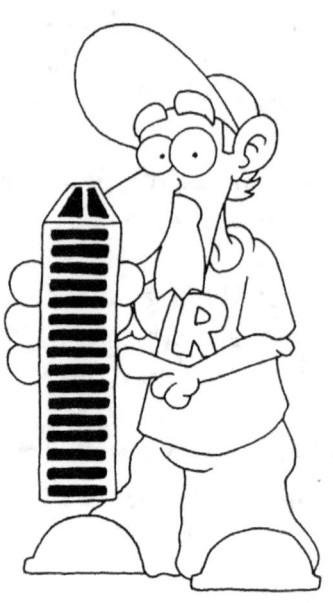

There's a lot of helpful information found on the food labels. If we are going to be buying it, we should at least take the time to learn about it. I mean, it's going to be in our bodies soon. You know what I mean?

The 5 Basic Food Groups

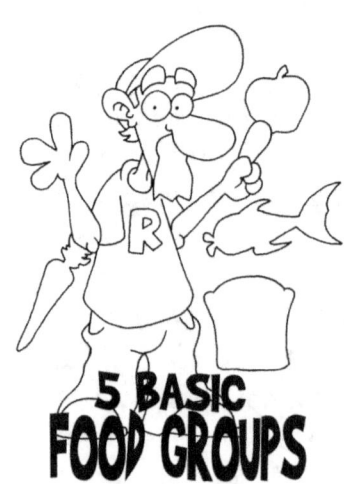

Remember learning about the 5 Basic Food Groups in school? Yeah, I know. It was a boring topic wasn't it? I bet we thought we would never need to know about this junk when we got older, huh? Wrong.

Basically, some smart folks got together and classified all of the food we eat into five basic groups. According to them, in order to live healthier, we should be eating something from each of these five groups every day.

Let's talk about them groups again. We'll call it a 'refresher' course. OK?

The Fruit Group
What is it? It's any fruit or 100% fruit juice. Fruits may be fresh, canned, frozen, or dried, and may be whole, cut-up, or pureed.

An apple is a fruit. A banana is a fruit. Bubble gum is not, even if it tastes like strawberries. You with me?

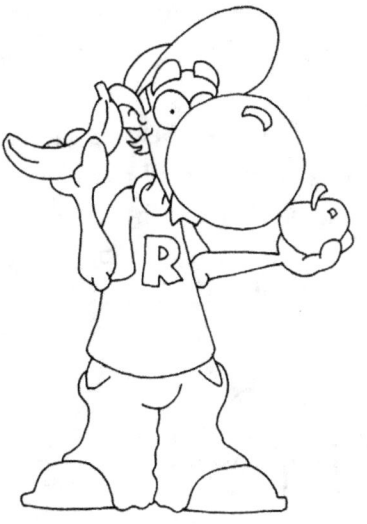

The Vegetable Group
What is it? It's any vegetable or 100% vegetable juice. Vegetables may be raw or cooked; fresh, frozen, canned, or dried/dehydrated; and may be whole, cut-up, or mashed.

Based on their nutrient content, vegetables are organized into 5 subgroups: dark green vegetables, starchy vegetables, red and orange vegetables, beans and peas, and other vegetables.

A potato is a vegetable, regardless if it's mashed, boiled, fried or served as a chip from a bag. It's still a potato. Catch that?

The Grain Group
What is it? It's any food made from wheat, rice, oats, cornmeal, barley or another cereal grain is a grain product. Bread, pasta, oatmeal, breakfast cereals, tortillas, and grits are examples of

grain products.

Grains are divided into 2 subgroups, Whole Grains and Refined Grains.

I know some of you don't know what a grit is. Yes, it's considered a Southern food and it is good for your health. Google it and find out where you can buy some. You can thank me later.

The Protein Foods Group

What is it? It's all foods made from meat, poultry, seafood, beans and peas, eggs, processed soy products, nuts, and seeds. Beans and peas are also part of the Vegetable Group. So, basically, if you double up on beans and peas throughout the day, it's OK.

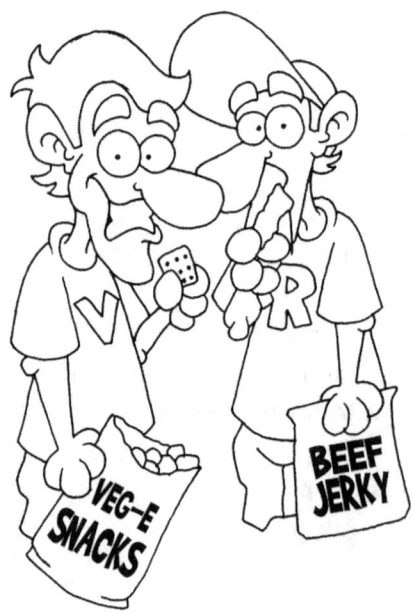

We all need protein for a healthy diet. Not everybody eats meat and that's OK. Vegetarians are still cool. For them, there are other foods that contain protein, such as nuts, seeds, beans and peas.

Unfortunately, you can't order any of them at a restaurant cooked Medium, Medium Well or Well Done. As my youngest daughter would say, "You get what you get, so don't pitch a fit."

The Dairy Group

What is it? It's all fluid milk products and many foods made from milk. Foods made from milk that retain their calcium content are part of the group. Foods made from milk that have little to no calcium, such as cream cheese, cream, and butter, are not. Calcium-fortified soymilk is also part of the Dairy Group.

Milk does your body good. It helps promote strong healthy bones and tastes great mixed in a bowl with cornbread. If you have never tried this, you should. It's also a Southern delicacy and makes a great late night snack.

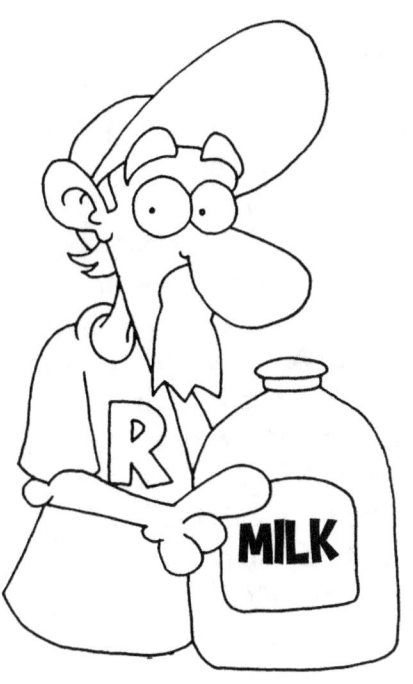

Improper Diet?
Look For The Signs

If we're not exercising or eating correctly, it will catch up with us one day because our body will let us know. You can count on it.

Here are some of those signs to look out for:

Size

The most obvious sign of a poor diet is that we either 'swell up like a whale' or 'become skinny as a rail'. When this happens, our clothes no longer fit. If we try to put on a pair of pants that we we wore last year and for some reason they don't fit, we should take a look at our diet. If your sweater appears to have shrunk since last winter, don't blame the clothes dryer or the husband that may have put it in there by mistake, check your diet first.

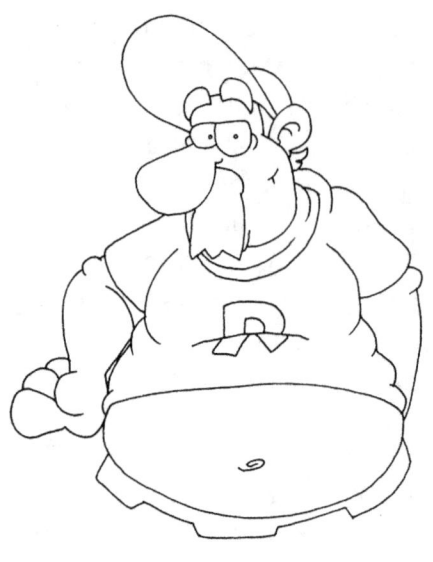

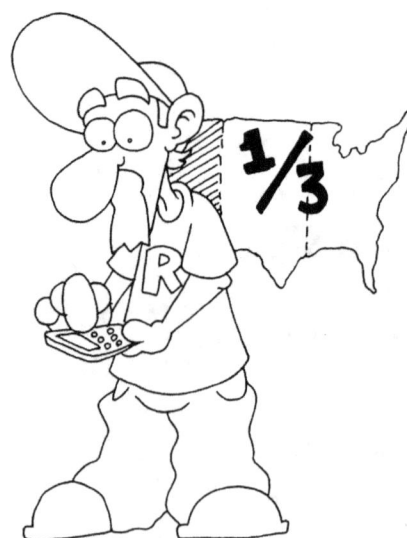

Has our eating habits changed? Are we still physically active? These are the questions we should ask ourselves.

The human body handles food energy pretty good. Whatever calories are not spent in exercise are stored in the form of fat. A person who eats less than they 'work off' becomes too thin, while someone who eats more than they burn becomes overweight.

Studies show that over one-third of American adults are overweight or obese. Wow! That's interesting.

Malnutrition

Someone who devours thousands of calories per day may not get the nutrition he needs for good health. If your diet consists of fast food take-out, you miss the essential vitamins and minerals found in fresh fruits and vegetables. The consequences are serious. For example, a vitamin A deficiency can cause blindness, while a vitamin C deficiency is responsible for a condition called scurvy, which results in dental problems.

Many of the toothless Redneck friends I know may not have dental hygiene problems after all. It could be from a Vitamin C deficiency. This would basically mean too much Mickey D and fatty cakes in their diet and not enough greens. You hear me?

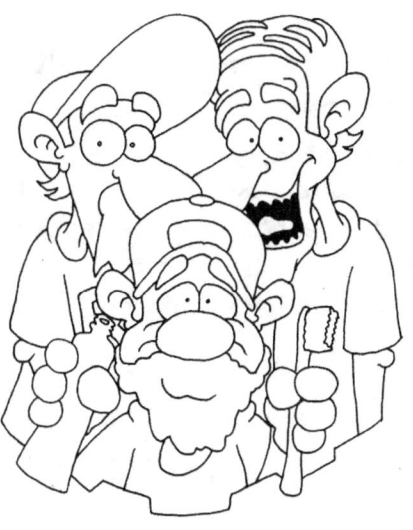

It's important to know that the foods we eat actually add value to our diets.

Fatigue

Not all food fuels are created the same. For example, the body burns through refined sugars very quickly which causes a condition called hypoglycemia. Try saying that word five times really fast.

If you eat foods made from refined sugars you get a sugar high, and when you crash from the sugar being burned up so quickly, it leaves you feeling worn out, light-headed and a little queasy. You end up with low blood sugar.

Anemia, or iron deficiency, is another reason people with a poor diet often feel tired and sluggish.

You know, maybe instead of boosting up on those energy drinks that leave you feeling 'crashed' later, we could simply eat better and healthier. That's a better idea!

Long Term Health Problems

There are a bunch of long term consequences of an improper diet. A few of the more serious physical side effects can be found on the next page.

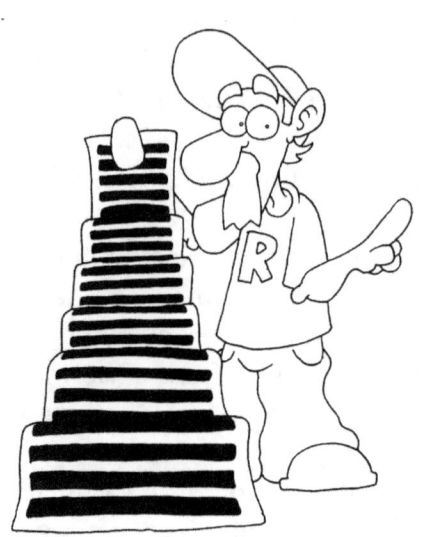

Effects Of Poor Nutrition On Your Health

If we keep on making poor choices when it comes to the food we eat, it can lead to a bunch of unhealthy outcomes.

I did some research and came up with a few. Here are some effects to the body from poor nutrition:

Cardiovascular disease (CVD): High blood cholesterol and lipid build-up can clog arteries, leading to cardiovascular disease. Fatty diets can lead to CVD.

Hypertension: Excessive sodium consumption and insufficient potassium in the diet can cause hypertension.

Diabetes: Diabetes occurs as a result of a metabolic disorder in the body. It can occur when the body does not make enough insulin to break down glucose (type 1 diabetes), or when the insulin present cannot be used (type 2 diabetes). Type 1 and 2 diabetes both lead to extreme amounts of blood glucose and medical problems. Type 1 diabetes is hereditary, but type 2 diabetes can occur as a result of obesity which is directly related to poor nutrition choices.

Cancer: In addition to genetics, dietary choices can affect the development of some cancers such as prostate cancer in men. Obese individuals are more prone to get prostate cancer.

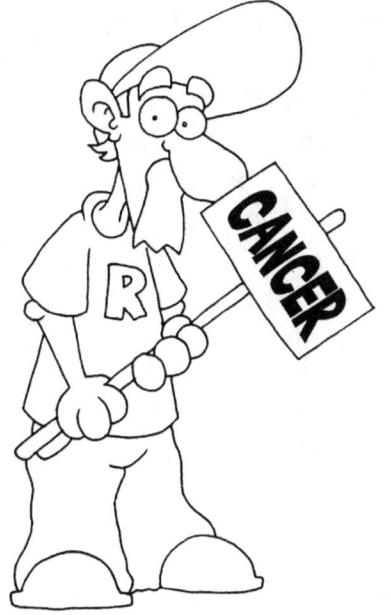

Osteoporosis: Osteoporosis-related fractures are as a result of inadequate nutrition and lack of physical activity.

Problems of being overweight or obese: Poor nutrition can cause individuals to be overweight or obese. Solutions such as decreasing sodium intake and calories from solid fats and added sugars can drastically reduce the occurrence of overweight or obesity health-related issues.

Mental Disorders: Poor nutrition can make certain mental illnesses worse. What you eat ultimately affects your emotions and proper brain functioning. Foods such as Omega-3 fatty acids affect neural functioning positively. A study done in Norway shows the connection between sugary soft drinks and mental health problems.

There's a price to pay for not eating correctly. We may not see it while we're young, but one day it will catch up with us. We will ultimately become what we eat. Every step we take now toward good health will help us to benefit from it when we get older. Think of it as an investment plan into our retirement.

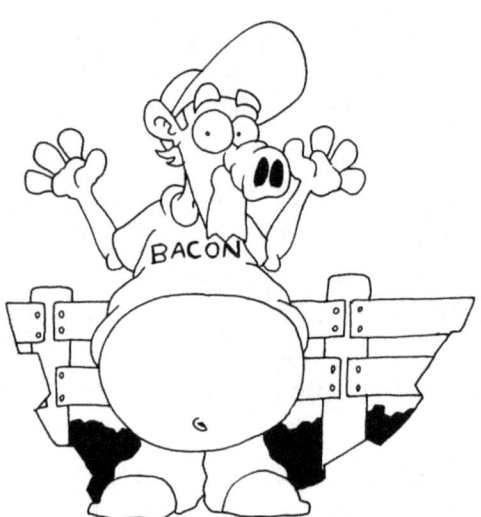

Some Reasons
For Poor Nutrition
With Simple Solutions

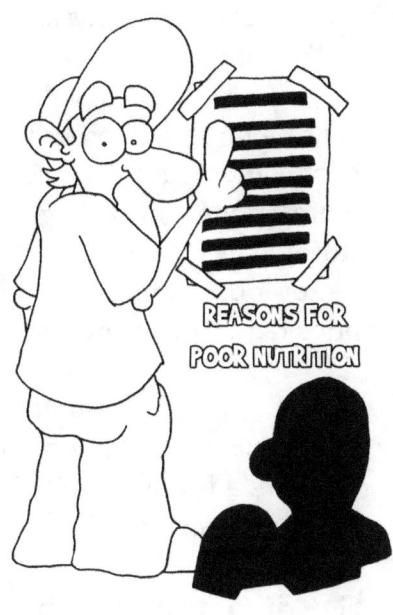

There are many reasons why people aren't eating healthy food. It would be great if we had the time, energy and resources to be able to provide our food from our own garden and farm because we know naturally fresh grown food from home is best for us. But, many of us don't. We may not have the luxury of owning acres of land with an endless supply of meat walking around the yard with four legs. Plus, for the folks living in subdivisions, there are rules about how we shouldn't have gardens and farm animals terrorizing the neighborhood. There are penalties to pay for breaking HOA rules and guidelines. So, what do you do? Well, you get it from the grocery store if you are able. Right?

If nutritious food is so easy to get from the grocery store, why would there be a problem with poor nutrition? Here are some of the reasons:

Poverty
Let's face it. Some people are too broke. Poverty and lack of

resources are two causes of bad nutrition that contribute to the estimated 925 million people worldwide suffering from the effects of malnutrition and the diseases that go along with it. The criteria for defining malnutrition are inadequate intake of protein and micronutrients, or vitamins and minerals, which causes millions of kids to die each year or to suffer lifelong physical and mental disabilities as the result of bad nutrition.

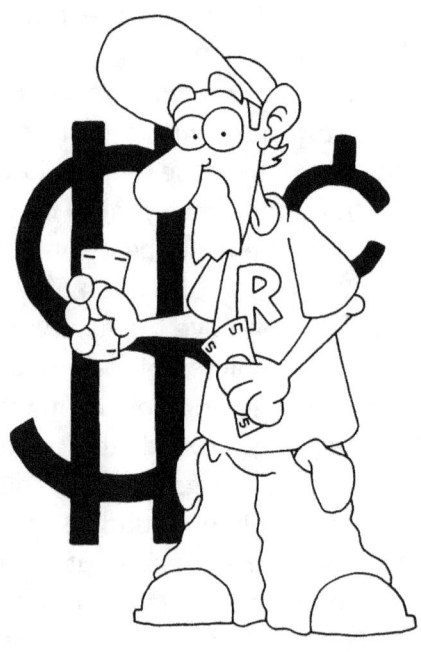

Let's be honest, in order to eat healthier, it's going to cost us more money at the grocery store. Right? It seems that the better foods come with higher price tags. Or do they?

Maybe its just a matter of rethinking the way we shop. Here are a few ways to help us cut our grocery bill:

Get rid of the junk food

We all love junk food. Most of the time we fill our buggies with it because it tastes so good. Yeah, we know its not good for our health, but we're willing to make the sacrifice.

Did you know that we could save a bunch of money if we cut out all of the junk food? These are foods that have very little nutritional value. This would include stuff like soda, cookies, crackers, prepackaged meals and processed foods. I know we all like those little single-packed fatty cakes that come in a box, but the money we could save could be used toward buying more healthier foods.

Make a grocery list and stick to it

I make lists. I usually start my day by creating a list of the things I want to accomplish for the day. The reason I do this is because my brain receives so many thoughts, ideas and distractions, that if I don't make a list, I wouldn't accomplish anything. It keeps me focused. Even though it sounds weird, it's actually not a bad idea if you are wanting to achieve goals. The brain can

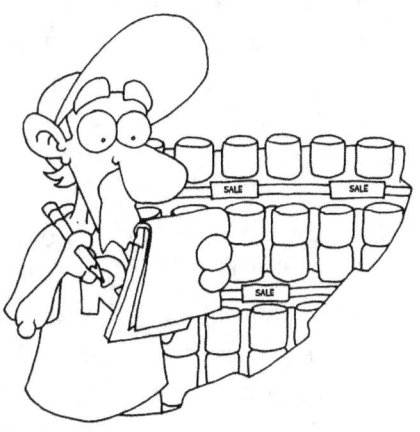

only hold so much information until it gets bombarded with so much stuff. The same applies when it comes to buying groceries.

Most people have a general idea of what they are wanting to get when they enter the grocery store. But, as soon as they get

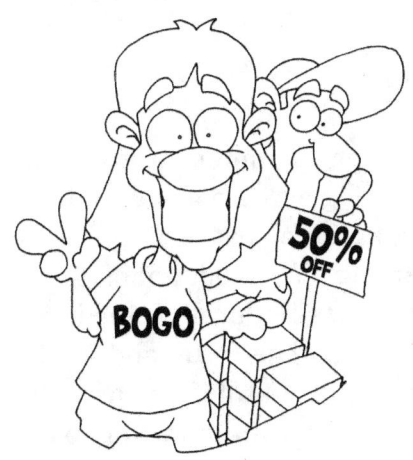

inside, they are distracted by all of the special deals, advertisements and things that pull their attention away from what they came in there to buy to begin with. But, if we knew what we were buying before we went to the grocery store, we could bypass all of these impulse purchases. Making a list could put more money back into our pocket.

My wife is guilty of being an impulse buyer. She won't admit it, but I know it's true. I dread it when she says that we are going shopping to buy 'one' item from the store. We have been married so long and from personal experience, I know that means we will walk out of that store with several bags.

For example, she will say, "We need to stop by Wally World. I need to get a gallon of milk."

That's sounds simple enough, right? It's not. The problem is that the gallon of milk is all the way across the store from the entrance door. As we proceed to get the milk, we will walk passed the produce section and she will pick up a bag of fruit. Then she will grab a loaf of bread. About midway through the store, she will notice a special on something for the house and she will put it in the buggy. All of a sudden she has to go to the bathroom, which is near the Electronics Department. She will pick up a movie and 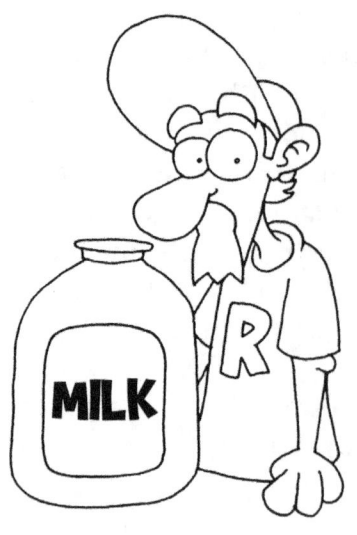 maybe some kind of accessory for her computer. At the same time, she will notice that they are having a clearance on clothing for our daughters, so she will stock up on all of the great deals. She will then catch a whiff of something that smells good coming from the area where the cleaning supplies are located. She might pick up a few things. Then, she regains her focus and begins walking towards the Dairy Section again. And before she grabs that gallon of milk, one of our girls will run over to the yogurt section and beg for us to buy them their favorite flavor with the cute cartoon character on the package. Finally, she gets the milk and we head toward the checkout counter. As we are standing in line, she remembers that she needs some hair coloring because we passed a mirror along the way and she saw some gray streaks on her head. We step out of line to walk all the way over to the hair products section. Of course, this is near the personal hygiene section. This area usually takes an hour because she has to sniff everything.

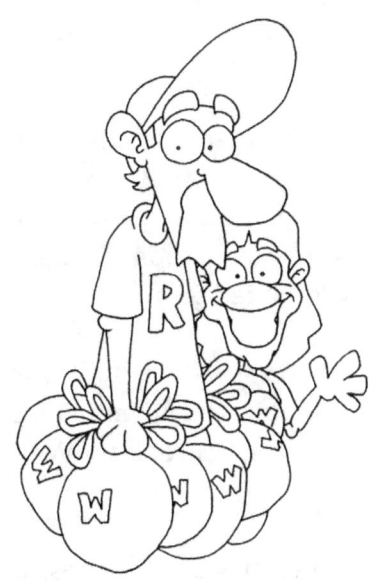

Three or four hours later, we are finally leaving the store. Our original plan of buying a gallon of milk has turned into an all day shopping frenzy. We are walking out of there with about ten bags of stuff and a receipt that is as tall as she is.

As we are loading the minivan with the bags, she says, "I need to make one more stop."

My head drops in silence because I realize my day is ruined.

Shop the outer edges of the store first

That's where most of the healthy food is located. It contains food such as fresh produce and meat. Most of what you see down the aisles is junk. When I say 'junk', I mean 'food' with no nutritional value. You could save some money by avoiding the inner aisles as much as possible.

Whether you knew it or not, stores are purposely laid out to maximize profits and make more money. This means it is designed to make us spend more money on junk. That could explain why the things we need are scattered all across the store. It forces us to look at all the other stuff, too.

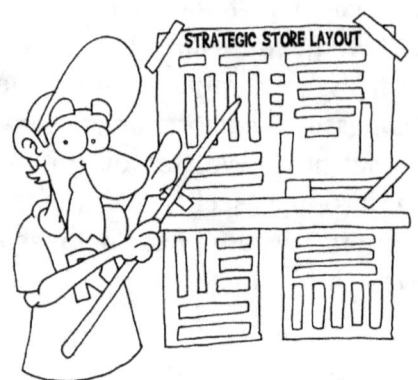

Have you ever wondered why most of the food products for kids are placed at the bottom level of the shelves? They want your child to see it. If they see it, they will beg and plead for you to buy it. To keep them quiet, we will usually put it in the buggy. The store just made a sale on something we may not have originally intended to buy.

We are being sold to. Most of the junk food stands out like a sore thumb down these aisles. We see it, we buy it and the store is happy. The whole marketing process was by their design. We are the victims.

We need to train ourselves to avoid the inner aisles if possible. Shop the outer edges first for healthier foods.

Cook in larger quantities

Instead of cooking one meal a day, you could cook enough for a couple of nights and store any extra in containers in the refrigerator. This is called 'having leftovers' and could save you money in the long run. If you know that you are cooking more at a time, you can buy food in bulk for a better savings.

My wife cooks soups and chili every now and then. The

48

ingredients she uses are affordable and she makes a bunch of it. In our house, a meal like this could last a couple of days. Based on our family size, we can save a good bit of money and it's healthier for our bodies.

Shop at discount stores

Places like Sam's Club, Costco Wholesale, BJ's Wholesale Club and many others offer discounts on stuff we eat from day to day. It's usually sold in bulk, so knowing how to proportion your meals and storing them wouldn't be a bad idea. A freezer then becomes a necessity.

Instead of having the mindset of buying 'once a week' or as a 'buy as you need it' basis, we could buy enough for the month on most food items. Discount stores could help and save us money when we buy in bulk.

Shop at Farmer's Markets

Most cities have them. It's where many local farmers get together and sell their goods to the general public. The prices offered are generally cheaper than what you can get from your grocery store.

Farmer's Markets are great because you can actually talk and learn about the one who grew your food personally. You can discover how they grew it and if chemicals were used. You can also negotiate pricing and work up some deals that you wouldn't normally be able to get at a grocery store.

If you aren't able to grow your own food, then a local farmer is the next best thing.

Buy generic and store brands

Most grocery stores have their own brand or some type of generic brand. This is the food that sits next to the major brand. You can always tell a store brand because the product label lacks color and is kinda dull looking. It could be just a white label with the name of the food typed on it. Store brands can sell for a cheaper price because there's no advertising expenses or marketing fees included. Most of the time generic or store brand food tastes about the same as the major brand.

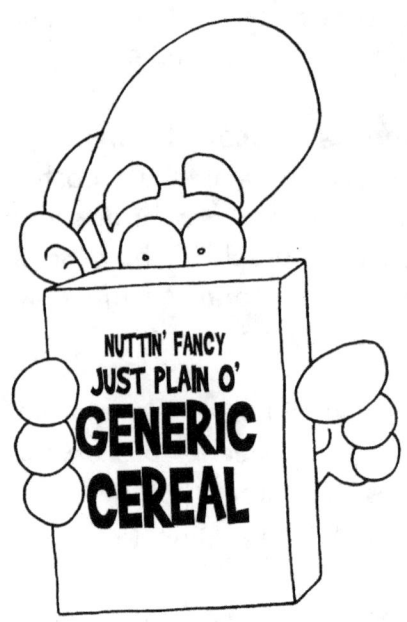

Because of media and the latest trends, we get caught up in all of the hoopla of what is considered popular. This affects the way we buy food. If we see it on a commercial, we automatically assume it is the best. Many times it is no better than a store brand item of the same thing. But, we buy it because we saw it on TV.

By buying generic or store brand, you can get more for your dollar. It's just a matter of changing the way you think and buy.

Limited Access

Studies show that bad nutrition is among the many factors contributing to childhood obesity. Basically, many kids are fat today because of the types of food they eat.

In some locations, access to supermarkets and large grocery stores is limited by distance, economic status and lack of transportation. People living in these areas, even though they can't get affordable nutritious food, they have easier access to fast foods that have very little nutritious value. This affects the daily nutritional needs of adults as well as children.

I believe this is true. It seems like there's a fast food restaurant around every corner. It's like gas stations. They're everywhere. Many times these fast food restaurants will even team up with these gas stations and join forces within the same building. Have you seen it? You stop by to get gas for your car on the way home from work and, at the same time, order a cheeseburger to go for dinner. It's kinda weird.

I live about 15 miles from town, but only a few miles from a McDoogle burger joint. If I were hungry and was limited on time, a cheeseburger is much easier to get and more convenient than

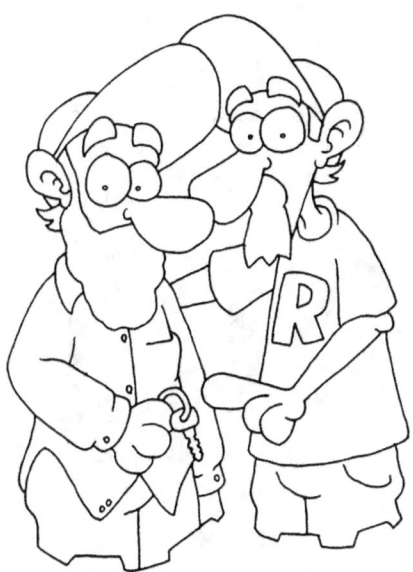

driving all the way across town to buy groceries. Many people feel this way, too.

For people that don't own a car or have a means of transportation, going to town could be impossible. In cases like this, it helps to have a friend, especially a friend with a car. Everybody has to have food, including neighbors. If transportation is a problem, a person could tag along with a friend or neighbor who is going to the grocery store anyway.

They could work together as a team and the money saved could be used towards the gas to get there.

This is where being 'social' goes beyond the Internet. We should get to know our neighbors and make friends with them on a personal level. We may need each other. The problem in the world today is that we stay so wrapped up in our own lives that we don't take the time to reach out to others that live on the same street. Many of us don't even know who our neighbors are. Families could save so much time and money if we shared our resources with one another.

Age-Related Nutrition Deficiency

Aging is an additional cause of bad nutrition. Older adults who live alone or have trouble getting around may have difficulty shopping for and preparing food. As a natural part of aging, changes that occur in taste and smell might cause a decrease in appetite, which leads to nutritional deficiencies. Economic hardship also contributes to the bad nutritional status of many senior citizens because it limits their food choices.

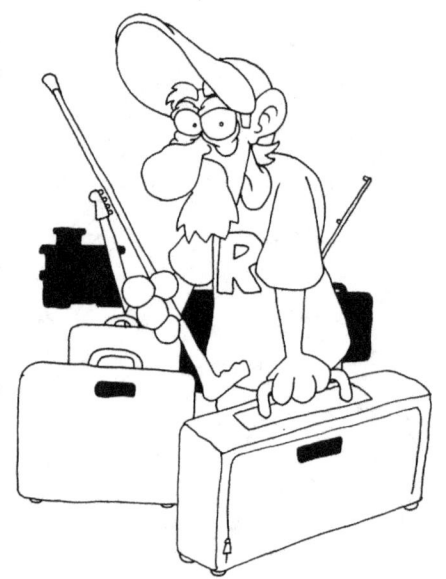

This is where having kids can help. We spend twenty years of our life helping our children to become able to stand on their own two feet. Now is the time that they should help us. It's how the family unit is supposed to work. We are to work together and help one another.

I make it a point to remind my kids why I am helping them. Yes, I am their parent and it is expected of me to do these things that I do, but I do expect a payback. When I am old, gray and can't take care of myself, I am packing my bags and moving in with them. I have already warned them. I have four kids and they better take turns or work together. It really doesn't matter to me how they do it as long as it happens. Just sayin'.

The fact is, family should help one another. We should take care of our elders when they aren't able. It's simply the right thing to do.

Social and Environmental Issues

Teenagers are known for making bad nutritional choices. They usually stick whatever they want in their mouths and call it food. It's usually the stuff that is quick and easy to make. Many adults are guilty of this, too.

A busy work or school schedule can make us eat more fast foods. We sometimes skip meals because we don't have time to eat. This is unhealthy because we starve our bodies of the proper nutrients that we need. This leads to health problems.

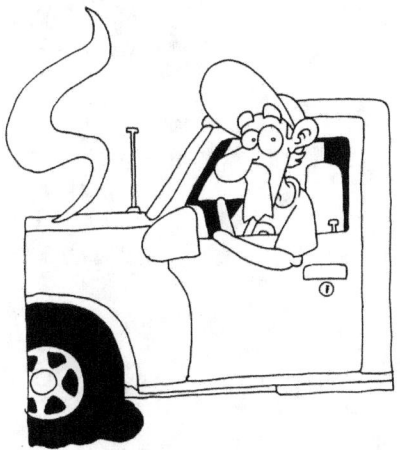

Eating correctly should be one of our main priorities every day. Our body's needs should be important. A busy life is like a car. Yes, there are many places that we think we need to go to, but without putting gas in it, how far will we actually go until it leaves us stranded on the side of the road? You know what I mean? We have to take care of our bodies.

Medications

Some over-the-counter and prescription medications affect the appetite and interfere with nutrient absorption and metabolism. People that take these medications over a long period of time could suffer from the same nutritional deficiencies as those who eat nutritionally poor diets.

We should talk with our doctors about any appetite problems that we notice. They should be able to help us to maintain a healthy balance. I, personally, wouldn't take it upon myself to get off of any medications without their consent. This could create some serious side effects. It's best to let them know so that they can find an alternate solution.

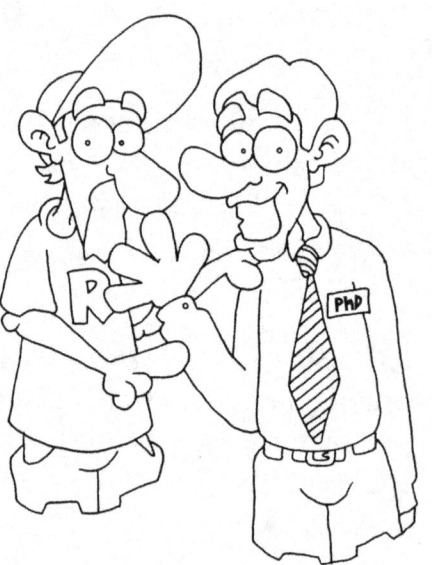

Exercise
Another Problem?

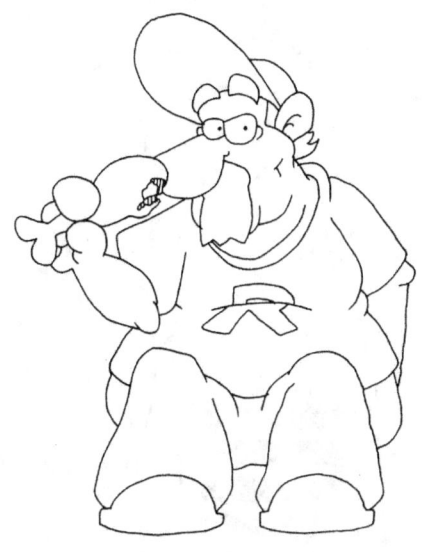

A lifestyle of 'sitting around all of the time doing nothing' is a common cause of obesity. All of this extra body weight and fat could 'open the door' and create more serious problems like diabetes, high blood pressure, joint damage and all kinds of other stuff.

This problem of 'not moving' not only affects the health of obese people, but also people of normal weight. These can be workers with desk jobs, people who are bed-ridden for a long period of time because of surgeries, injuries and complications with pregnancy. Going without exercise does damage to the the body (structurally and metabolically). It can cause the heart rate to 'go through the roof' during physical activity, our bones and muscles can waste away and deteriorate, our physical endurance can 'bottom out' quickly and cause our blood volume to decline.

Several serious medical conditions are associated with a lack of exercise, including fibromyalgia, chronic fatigue syndrome and postural orthostatic tachycardia syndrome (POTS). POTS is a syndrome marked by an excessive heart rate and flu-like symptoms when standing or a given level of exercise. Many times medication, instead of exercise, is prescribed.

What if many of the health problems we have today could be fixed by simply exercising? A few minutes of movement is a whole lot better than popping pills every day. You agree?

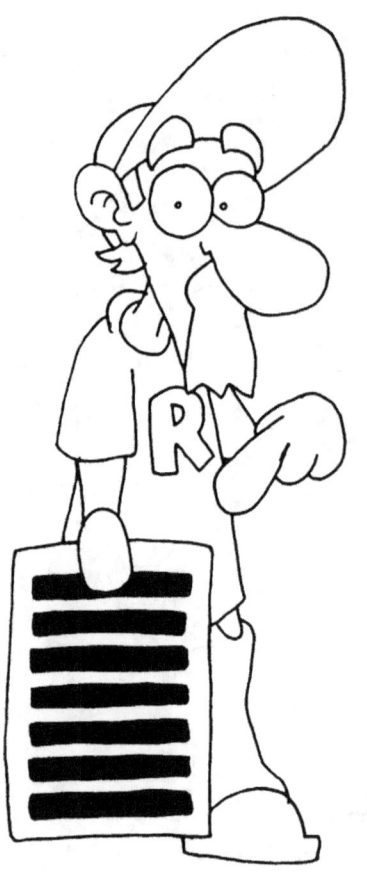

Lack Of Exercise
It's Effect On The Body

Exercise has a lot of benefits. It helps us keep off excess weight. It makes our bones strong. It also keeps our heart healthy.

On the flipside, not exercising can have an opposite effect on our health. It can make our bones weak, cause our organs to malfunction and cause us to gain weight. Gaining weight could lead to other obesity-related medical conditions, such as diabetes or hypertension.

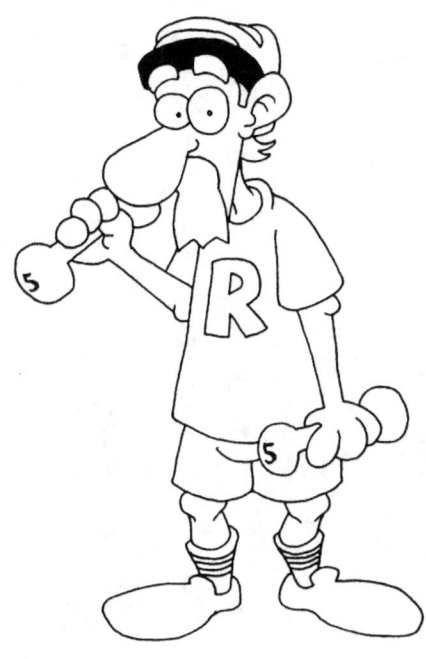

Here are some medical conditions created from lack of exercise:

Muscle Atrophy

Muscle atrophy is the medical term that describes the process of your muscles wasting away. When your muscles aren't exercised to their full capacity, they begin to break down. Not only does this cause you lose lean muscle mass, but it also causes fatty tissue to develop around your muscles. Muscle burns fat, so when your body doesn't have much muscle, your metabolism slows, and you begin to gain weight.

Cardiac Decline

Lack of exercise can also cause fatty deposits to develop around your heart and in your arteries. Fatty deposits can also enter the valves and chambers of your heart, which can lead to heart failure or a heart attack. A study showed that approximately 2.4 million Americans died from heart disease in 2006. Heart disease is still one of the leading causes of death in America.

Increased Visceral Fat

Visceral fat is fat that becomes entrapped deep inside your

abdomen. It surrounds your heart and other organs and can cause a multitude of health problems, including heart disease, gallbladder problems, metabolic syndrome and a whole lot more. This fat also secretes dangerous hormones. Some of the hormones produced by these fat cells can increase your risk of developing breast cancer and promote insulin resistance, which might lead to diabetes.

Intestinal Effects

Lack of exercise can also cause constipation. Exercise promotes digestion and helps your body pass solid waste. When you don't exercise, your body's digestion process slows down. If you have a lot of visceral fat and irregular bowel movements, your risk of developing colorectal cancer increases. Exercising regularly to keep your weight under control and increasing the amount of fiber in your diet can lower your risk of developing this cancer. To put it 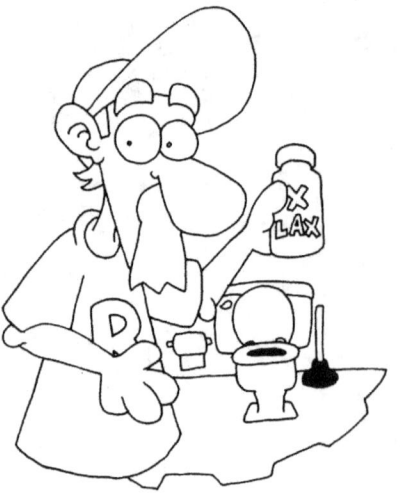 into simple terms, exercise helps you poop, keeps you regular and lowers your risk of getting health problems.

Regular physical activity is one of the most important things you can do for your health. It can help:

- Control your weight
- Lower your risk of heart disease
- Lower your risk for type 2 diabetes and metabolic syndrome

- Lower your risk of some cancers
- Strengthen your bones and muscles
- Improve your mental health and mood
- Improve your ability to do daily activities and prevent falls, if you're an older adult
- Increase your chances of living longer

Fitting regular exercise into your daily schedule may seem hard to do at first. But even ten minutes at a time is OK. The key is to find the right exercise for you. It should be fun and should match your abilities.

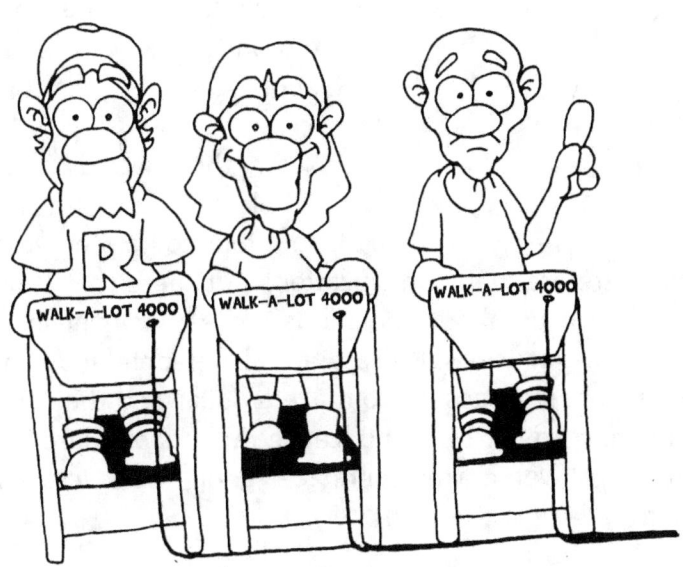

What Does The Bible Say?

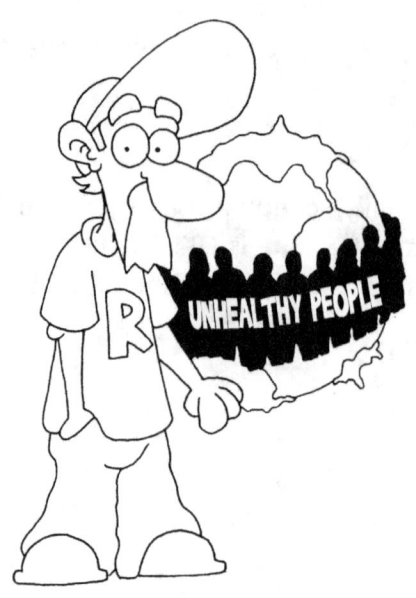

There are issues in the world today with the food we eat and problems created from our lack of exercise. No doubt! Many people walking around today are unhealthy and dying because of it. The sad thing is that it's a slow death. We may start by eating unhealthy as a child and not see the side effects from it until we are too old and wrinkly to do anything about it.

Yes, the world sees the problems and has many solutions to help prevent it and treat it. There are many organizations out there that step out to help and warn us about the foods we eat or explain why it's important to exercise. But, there are also people and companies out there whose purpose is to make a dollar and they don't care who they hurt to get it. And because most people are lazy, they buy into whatever makes them feel good, work less and save money. It's just how the world turns.

The Bible tells us that 'the love of money is the root of all evil'. Living unhealthy and dying younger than we should wasn't part of God's original plan for society. He wants us all to prosper and live life to it's fullest. God is love and wants the very best for all of us.

He that loveth not knoweth not God; for God is love. In this was manifested the love of God toward us, because that God sent his only begotten Son into the world, that we might live through him. - 1 John 4: 8, 9

The thief cometh not, but for to steal, and to kill, and to destroy: I am come that they might have life, and that they might have it more abundantly. - John 10: 10

God created us and has provided us with the food we need to survive. He provided the animals for us to eat. He gave us the seed, soil, water and sun to grow the vegetables and fruit for us to eat, too.

Everything we need to know can be found in the Bible. God has already placed a Food Plan in motion and it can be found in the Old Testament. It is part of the laws that God provided Moses as they journeyed to the Promised Land.

Keep in mind, as Christians, we are not bound to the laws mentioned in the Old Testament. We are saved by faith in Jesus Christ.

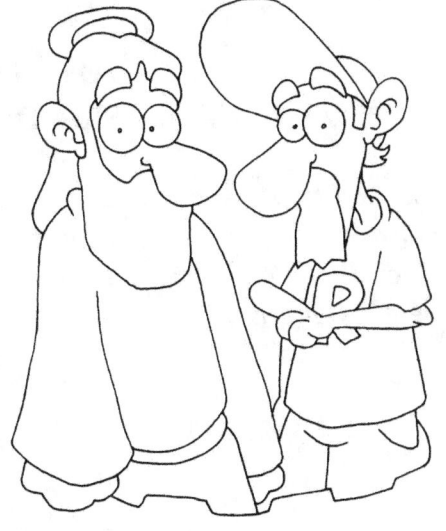

Knowing that a man is not justified by the works of the law, but by the faith of Jesus Christ, even we have believed in Jesus Christ, that we might be justified by the faith of Christ, and not by the works of the law: for by the works of the law shall no flesh be justified. - Galatians 2: 16

What that means is that we're not saved by following the laws of the Old Testament. We are saved by having faith in Jesus. However, the laws were written and designed to help us live better and we can use them to improve our lifestyle. Eating pork (which is forbidden to eat according to the law) will not send you to eternity in a lake of fire. However, by eating it, it could create some health problems. You see what I'm saying? These laws are there to help us. God wrote them.

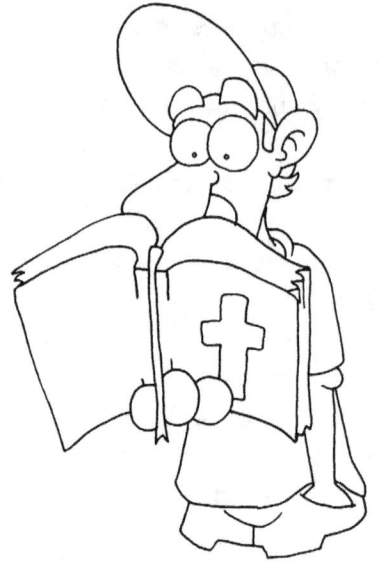

Let's read them to see what He has to say.

God's Plan
Vegetables – Side Dish or Main Course

And God said, Behold, I have given you every herb bearing seed, which is upon the face of all the earth, and every tree, in the which is the fruit of a tree yielding seed; to you it shall be for meat. - Genesis 1: 29

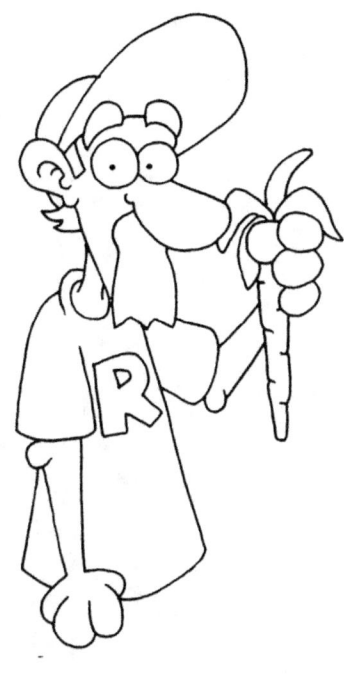

The world contains all of the food we need. God put it there for us since the very beginning.

If you think about all of the vegetables and fruits we eat that we grow or buy from the grocery store, it originated from God. He invented it. In His awesome perfect plan, He has given us a rainbow assortment of nutrition to help us stay healthier and live better.

All that we eat has color. Every fruit and vegetable is unique in its own way. Tomatoes are red. Lemons are yellow. Broccoli is green. Have you ever wondered why? Each offers its own special attribute to our health.

I learned that the more colors of food you put on your dinner plate, the more healthier your meal will be. That makes sense and its by God's design.

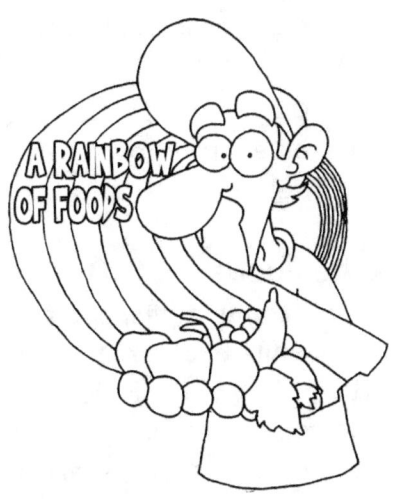

Let's take a closer look at God's Rainbow of food:

Red Foods
Trees: cherries, apples, cranberries, papaya, pomegranate

Plants: tomatoes, strawberries, watermelon, raspberries
Herbs: beets, rhubarb, radishes

Orange Foods
Trees: oranges, grapefruit, peaches
Plants: pumpkin, squash
Herbs: carrots, sweet potatoes, yams

Yellow Foods
Trees: lemons, pears, apricots, grapefruit
Plants: corn, squash, wheat, cantaloupe
Herbs: rutabagas

Green Foods
Trees: avocados, olives, pears, lime
Plants: cucumbers, peas, green beans, zucchini
Herbs: broccoli, asparagus, greens, spinach, brussels sprouts, kale, celery, green onions

Blue Foods
Plants: blueberries, blackberries, mulberries

White Foods
Trees: coconut, dates, pears, nuts
Plants: white beans, oats
Herbs: onions, cauliflower, garlic, horseradish, potatoes, turnips, mushrooms, parsnips, shallots, ginger

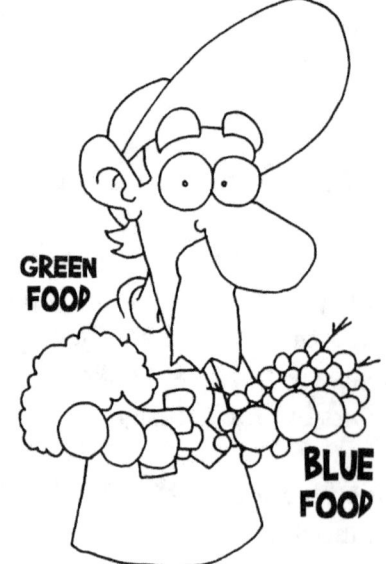

GREEN FOOD

BLUE FOOD

Purple Foods

Trees: plums, prunes, figs
Plants: grapes, blackberries, elderberries
Herbs: beets, eggplants, cabbage

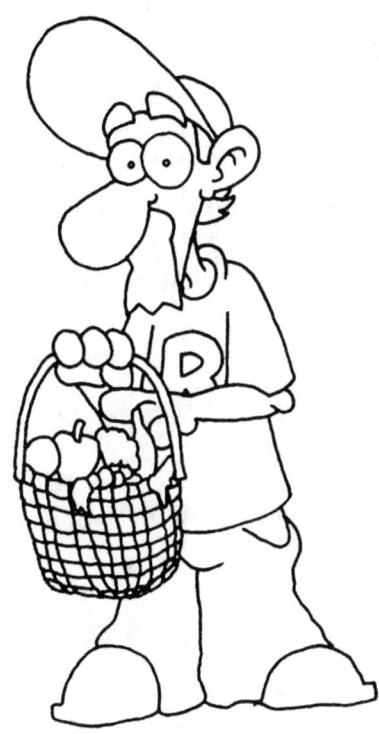

All of these foods are great to eat and they are good for our bodies. It's awesome to know that God took the time to create each one – the taste, color and texture. He could have just made a plain gray fruit or vegetable and been done. But, no! He made something beautiful for us to enjoy with all of our senses.

By eating something from every color, you would be adding nutritious value to your diet and your health.

God's Plan
Meat – The Main Entree

Ye are the children of the LORD your God: ye shall not cut yourselves, nor make any baldness between your eyes for the dead. For thou art an holy people unto the LORD thy God, and the LORD hath chosen thee to be a peculiar people unto himself, above all the nations that are upon the earth. Thou shalt not eat any abominable thing. - Deuteronomy 14: 1 – 3

And the LORD spake unto Moses and to Aaron, saying unto them, Speak unto the children of Israel, saying, These are the beasts which ye shall eat among all the beasts that are on the earth. - Leviticus 11: 1, 2

God wanted to create a great nation that was special to Him – Israel. He provided them with laws, not to create servants, slaves and mindless sheeple, but to build a nation that was holy and above all nations. He loved them and wanted what was best for them – physically and spiritually.

The same applies to each of us today.

A new heart also will I give you, and a new spirit will I put within you: and I will take away the stony heart out of your flesh, and I will give you an heart of flesh.
And I will put my spirit within you, and cause you to walk in my statutes, and ye shall keep my judgments, and do them. And ye shall dwell in the land that I gave to your fathers; and ye shall be my people, and I will be your God. - Ezekiel 36: 26-28

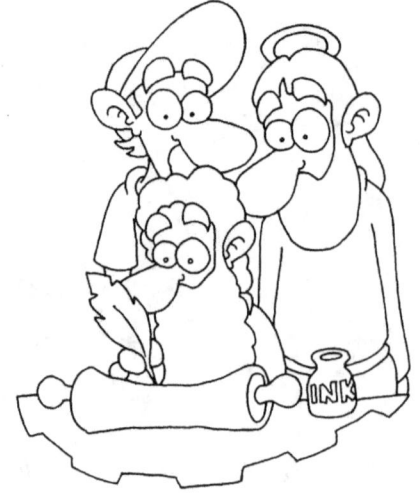

To create this special nation under God, the laws included a special dietary plan. God knew His creation and designed certain animals for human consumption.

All flesh is not the same flesh: but there is one kind of flesh of men, another flesh of beasts, another of fishes, and another of birds. - 1 Corinthians 15: 39

I imagine eating any thing, other than what God allowed in His law, could have some negative side effects. This could possibly explain why we have a growing issue with health problems in the world today.

Meat - Of The Earth

These are the beasts which ye shall eat: the ox, the sheep, and the goat, The hart, and the roebuck, and the fallow deer, and the wild goat, and the pygarg, and the wild ox, and the chamois. And every beast that parteth the hoof, and cleaveth the cleft into two claws, and cheweth the cud among the beasts, that ye shall eat. Nevertheless these ye shall not eat of them that chew the cud, or of them that divide the cloven hoof; as the camel, and the hare, and the coney: for they chew the cud, but divide not the hoof; therefore they are unclean unto you. And the swine, because it divideth the hoof, yet cheweth not the cud, it is unclean unto you: ye shall not eat of their flesh, nor touch their dead carcase. - Deuteronomy 14: 4 – 8

Whatsoever parteth the hoof, and is clovenfooted, and cheweth the cud, among the beasts, that shall ye eat. Nevertheless these shall ye not eat of them that chew the cud, or of them that divide the hoof: as the camel, because he cheweth the cud, but divideth not the hoof; he is unclean unto you. And the coney, because he cheweth the cud, but divideth not the hoof; he is unclean unto you. And the hare, because he cheweth the cud, but divideth not the hoof; he is unclean unto you. And the swine, though he divide the hoof, and be clovenfooted, yet he cheweth not the cud; he is unclean to you. Of their flesh shall ye not eat, and their carcase shall ye not touch; they are unclean to you.- Leviticus 11: 3 - 8

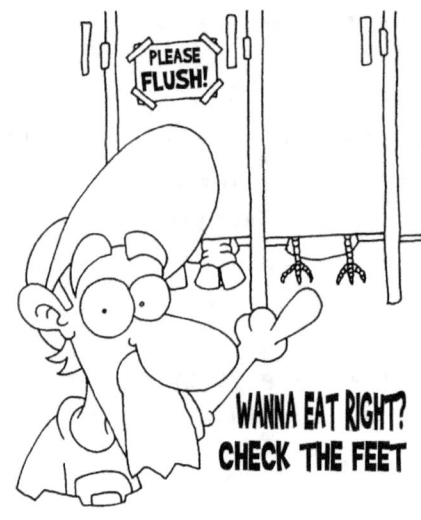

PLEASE FLUSH!

WANNA EAT RIGHT?
CHECK THE FEET

According to the law, land animals that have a split hoof divided in two and that chews the cud were acceptable to eat. This would involve looking at an animal's feet and checking out their dinner menu. The term 'chewing the cud' is basically what certain animals do when they have more than one stomach. It's kinda gross, but what happens is that the food that they partially chew goes into one stomach and then it's puked up and chewed again. Yeah, I told you it was gross.

The process breaks the food down and allows the animal to receive more of its nutrients. If the animal doesn't 'chew the cud' or if it is fed the wrong kind of food, it will get sick and possibly become diseased. This disease may become part of the food we eat. Ever heard of Mad Cow Disease? It's believed by some that it could come from the kind of food that a cow was allowed to eat.

What animals are considered 'cud chewers'? The Bible includes ox, sheep, goat, deer, gazelle, ibex and antelope. Additional animals that are OK to eat based on the law's criteria include buffalo, cattle, rams, elks, moose, caribou and giraffes. The exceptions that could not be eaten according to the Bible include the camel, rabbit, pig and coney (which is a type of rabbit or rodent).

If you learn more about the different types of meat that we buy from the grocery store, you discover that our health is potentially at risk. In many cases, meat is injected with all kinds of chemicals and the animals are fed stuff that isn't natural. Their living conditions are inhumane. If we saw what these animals went through before they became food on our dinner plate, it would probably make us all become vegetarians.

The Food Law from the Bible was written based on naturally raised animals. It took into consideration what an animal ate in natural situations. Their diet was the criteria used to determine if they were considered 'clean' or 'unclean' for our human consumption.

An example would be a pig. We all know pigs eat 'slop' and basically eat anything you feed it. They are known to have worms and parasites. They don't sweat to remove any impurities in their body. It would be considered 'unclean' because we would be eating all of this junk, too.

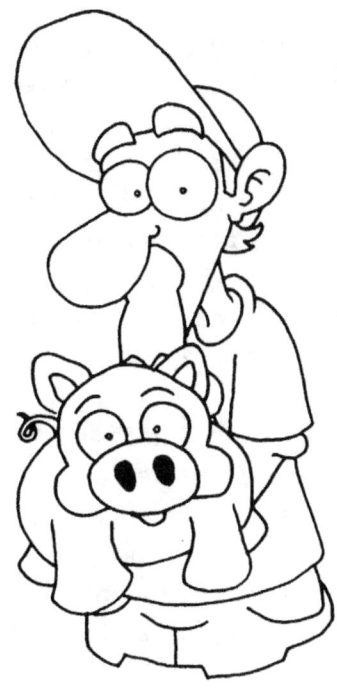

A rabbit was considered 'unclean', too. Why? I mean, these animals eat healthy. They hop around all day eating grass, carrots and lay eggs at Easter, right? They are considered 'lean' and high in protein. What could possibly be wrong with eating a rabbit? Studies show that eating foods that are too high in protein can actually kill you. It's called 'protein poisoning' or 'rabbit starvation'. The human body has to have a well-balanced diet of nutrients from fats, proteins, carbohydrates, water, vitamins and minerals. Some meats just don't supply it. The hard work of discovering which meats are good for us and which ones are not has already been done in the Bible. God did it for us.

On a personal note, I am glad that a deer made the list of 'clean' food. Rednecks, like myself, love deer meat. Am I right?

Meat - Of The Water

These ye shall eat of all that are in the waters: all that have fins and scales shall ye eat: And whatsoever hath not fins and scales ye may not eat; it is unclean unto you. - Deuteronomy 14: 9, 10

These shall ye eat of all that are in the waters: whatsoever hath fins and scales in the waters, in the seas, and in the rivers, them shall ye eat. And all that have not fins and scales in the seas, and in the rivers, of all that move in the waters, and of any living thing which is in the waters, they shall be an abomination unto you: They shall be even an abomination unto you; ye shall not eat of their flesh, but ye shall have their carcases in abomination. Whatsoever hath no fins nor scales in the waters, that shall be an abomination unto you. - Leviticus 11: 9 - 12

The Food Law states that the only creatures living in the water that could be eaten were fish that had fins and scales. This would include trout, tuna fish, salmon, halibut, bluegills, sunfish, cod fish, flounder, perch, herring, sardines, bass, smelt and mackerels. The exceptions that could not be eaten were fish that did not have fins and scales.

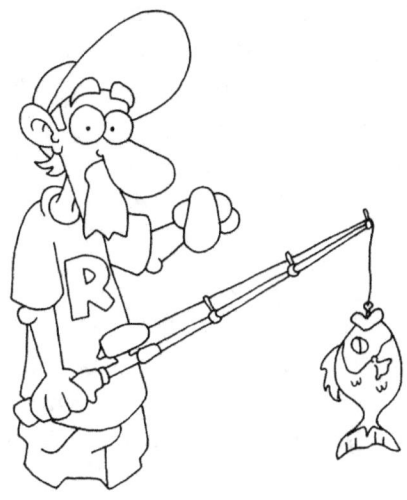

Let's think about that for a minute. What kind of fish do we currently eat that does and does not have fins? We probably don't think much about it. We basically just 'eat fish' because we are told by professionals that all fish are good for us. Right? Plus, if we buy fish from the grocery store, most of the time it has been de-finned and de-scaled. So, how will we know? This will take doing some research on our part.

Here are some of the commonly known fish that we eat:

Fish with no scales - shellfish, shrimp, catfish, lobster, mussels, eels, sharks, sturgeons, and swordfish. This is just a few of them. According to the Food Laws in the Bible, we shouldn't eat these.

Fish with scales - albacore, bass, carp, flounder, grouper, haddock, halibut, herring, mackerel, mahi mahi, orange roughy, perch, pike, pollock, salmon, sardines, snapper, sole, tilapia, trout, tuna, walleye, whitefish and whiting. According to the Food Laws in the Bible, these are good for us.

From what I've learned, the main difference in fish with scales and fish without scales is their digestive systems. Why would this be a problem? Well, the digestive system in a fish with fins and scales prevents the absorption of poisons and toxins into their flesh that they get from the waters that they swim in.

This is sad news for me because I love eating catfish and shrimp.

Don't we all? I learned that catfish are scavengers that feed off the bottom of the water and their digestive system is designed to absorb toxins from the water. Their purpose would be to help keep the waters clean and not part of our menu. This would make them a potential health hazard for us if we chose to eat them.

Clams, lobster, shrimp, crabs, mussels and squid do not have scales or fins and are believed to be highly toxic. They naturally absorb all of the toxins in the water. Believe it or not, lobster and crabs are crustaceans and are a part of the arthropod family, which include creatures like caterpillars, cockroaches, and spiders! Yeah, I didn't know that either.

It seems that most of the seafood we enjoy eating is bad for us according to the Bible. It makes me wonder if, somewhere down the line, someone changed things.

Maybe a bunch of fishermen got tired of having to throw back all of the 'unclean' fish into the water and said, "Hey! It sure is a lot of hard work having to throw all of these bad fish back. It's making my back hurt. Let's keep them and sell them instead. Hey! People don't pay much attention to what they eat anyway. We could make millions."

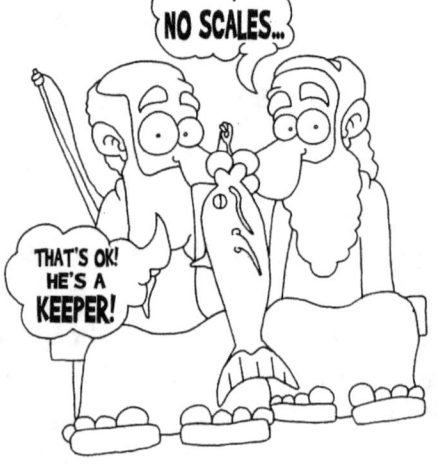

And the seafood business exploded.

Meat - Of The Air

Of all clean birds ye shall eat. But these are they of which ye shall not eat: the eagle, and the ossifrage, and the ospray, And the glede, and the kite, and the vulture after his kind, And every raven after his kind, And the owl, and the night hawk, and the cuckow, and the hawk after his kind, The little owl, and the great owl, and the swan, And the pelican, and the gier eagle, and the cormorant, And the stork, and the heron after her kind, and the lapwing, and the bat. -Deuteronomy 14: 11 – 18

And these are they which ye shall have in abomination among the fowls; they shall not be eaten, they are an abomination: the eagle, and the ossifrage, and the ospray, And the vulture, and the kite after his kind; Every raven after his kind; And the owl, and the night hawk, and the cuckow, and the hawk after his kind, And the little owl, and the cormorant, and the great owl, And the swan, and the pelican, and the gier eagle, And the stork, the heron after her kind, and the lapwing, and the bat. All fowls that creep, going upon all four, shall be an abomination unto you.- Leviticus 11: 13 - 19

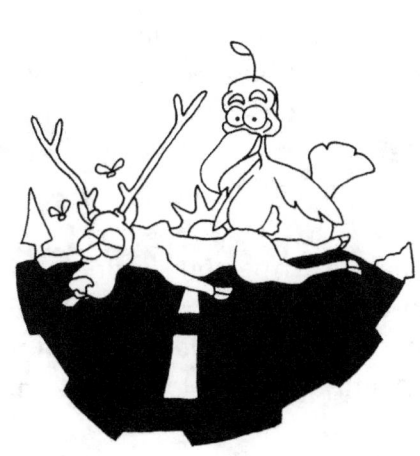

According to the Food Law, people could only eat 'clean' birds. This would include animals such as chickens, turkeys, partridges, sparrows, doves, pheasants and quail. The exceptions that could not be eaten were eagles, vultures, kites, falcons, ravens, owls, ospreys, cormorants, storks, herons, hoopoes, and bats.

Here again, the difference is in

the bird's digestive system and what it eats that makes it 'clean' or 'unclean'. A bird that you see in the middle of the street eating 3-day old roadkill would be a health risk if you ate it because of the bacteria and junk in its digestive system.

I am just glad that chicken and turkey made the 'clean' list. These are affordable meats at the grocery store. And you know how us Rednecks just love chicken!

Meat – The Creeping Things

And every creeping thing that flieth is unclean unto you: they shall not be eaten. But of all clean fowls ye may eat. - Deuteronomy 14: 19, 20

Yet these may ye eat of every flying creeping thing that goeth upon all four, which have legs above their feet, to leap withal upon the earth; Even these of them ye may eat; the locust after his kind, and the bald locust after his kind, and the beetle after his kind, and the grasshopper after his kind. But all other flying creeping things, which have four feet, shall be an abomination unto you. - Leviticus 11: 20 - 23

According to the Food Law, you could eat any winged creature that is clean and must have four legs and hop. Some examples would include grasshoppers, locusts, crickets and katydids. The exceptions that could not be eaten would be all flying insects that swarm. This would include bees and flies.

This is a funny category for me because I personally don't eat bugs unless I'm driving in my Jeep with the top down and I have my mouth open. Eating bugs in this case would be by pure accident. I don't find them a bit appetizing at all. However, some folks do. Hey! Whatever rocks your boat!

Many bugs carry toxins that are considered unhealthy if we decide to eat them. On the other hand, grasshoppers, locusts and crickets have been proven to be an alternate source of protein and are actually good for you. Yes, people actually eat them.

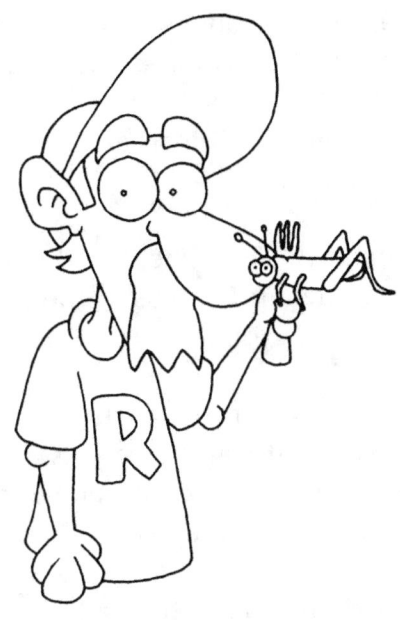

One of the things I found interesting is that we are actually eating bugs from day to day and don't even know it. Say what?

Yep! It's true! Believe it or not,

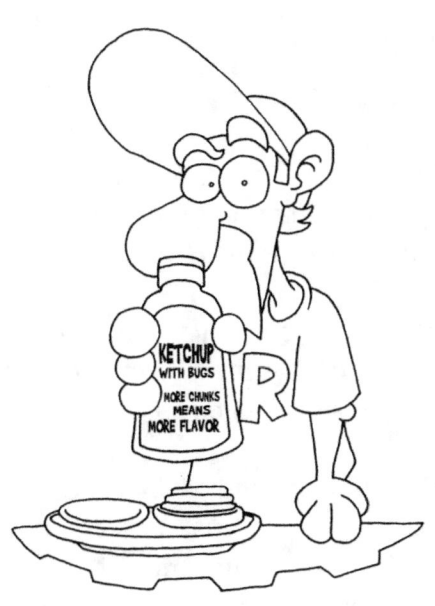

bugs are in the foods we eat. If we think about how food is produced, manufactured and passed through assembly lines, the chances of bugs falling into the whole process is pretty good. Actually, the U.S. FDA allows a certain amount of bugs to be in there because its impossible to prevent it. They don't tell you this in the ingredients. This is covered up by food coloring and bleaching. This can't be good for our health.

Can you imagine what would happen if ketchup included bugs in its ingredients on the label? I can see it now.

"Ingredients: Tomatoes, corn syrup, vinegar, salt, roaches, flies and beetles"

I don't think people would buy it. Do you? It looks better when they cover it up by using the word 'Natural Flavors'. It just sounds more appetizing.

God has a purpose for the Food Laws found in Deuteronomy and Leviticus. It wasn't just a list of rules that He expected everyone to follow. It was a guideline to healthy living that He wrote out of His love for humanity.

We should take it to heart.

God's Plan
Exercise

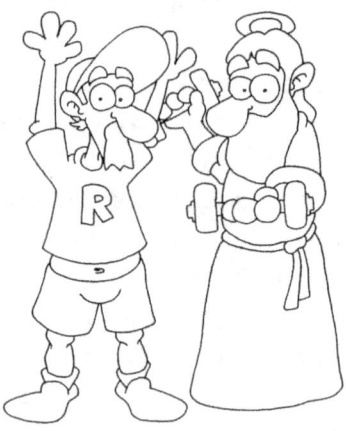

How long wilt thou sleep, O sluggard? when wilt thou arise out of thy sleep? - Proverbs 6:9

And whatsoever ye do, do it heartily, as to the Lord, and not unto men; - Colossians 3: 23

Even though the Bible doesn't specifically give us an exercise program like doing fifty jumping jacks every day or ten situps every three hours, it does recognize the value of exercise. But mostly, it emphasizes the importance of living according to God's Word and treating it as our top priority in life.

For bodily exercise profiteth little: but godliness is profitable unto all things, having promise of the life that now is, and of that which is to come. - 1 Timothy 4: 8

Most of what you read about physical activity in the Bible is mentioned by the term 'work'. People worked the land to produce their food. People worked physically in order to build, grow and do the things they needed to do from day to day. They didn't have modern day conveniences to do the work for them like we do today. It was all physical.

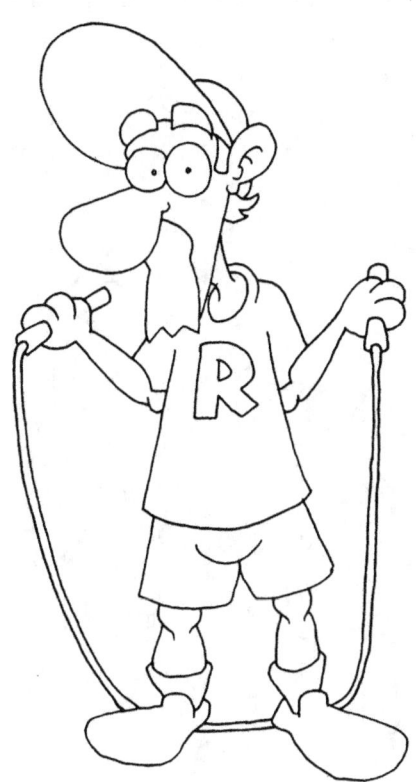

And unto Adam he said, Because thou hast hearkened unto the voice of thy wife, and hast eaten of the tree, of which I commanded thee, saying, Thou shalt not eat of it: cursed is the ground for thy sake; in sorrow shalt thou eat of it all the days of thy life; Thorns also and thistles shall it bring forth to thee; and thou shalt eat the herb of the field; In the sweat of thy face shalt thou eat bread, till thou return unto the ground; for out of it wast thou taken: for dust thou art, and

77

unto dust shalt thou return. - Genesis 3: 17-19

Hard work was a curse placed on mankind for man's disobedience to God in the very beginning. However, the reward for hard work is the satisfaction of actually doing something constructive and being able to eat 'from the sweat of your brow'.

In the sweat of thy face shalt thou eat bread, till thou return unto the ground; for out of it wast thou taken: for dust thou art, and unto dust shalt thou return. - Genesis 3: 19

This is really how life goes. We work, we eat and eventually die. Of course, we do get to enjoy stuff along the way.

For even when we were with you, this we commanded you, that if any would not work, neither should he eat. - 2 Thessalonians 3: 10

There is a lot mentioned in the Bible about being lazy and how it's not good to be this way. God wants us to be moving and doing something constructive.

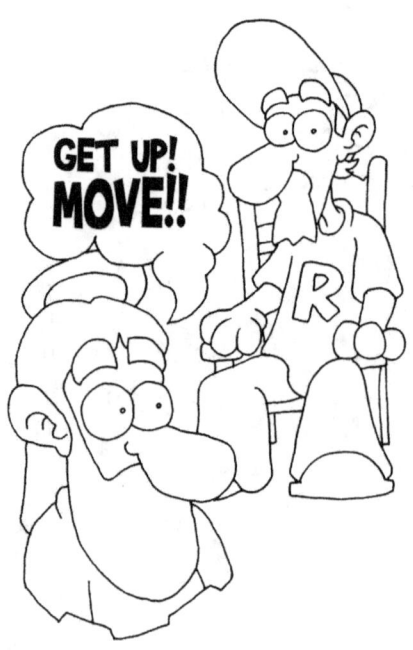

Go to the ant, thou sluggard; consider her ways, and be wise: - Proverbs 6: 6

The desire of the slothful killeth him; for his hands refuse to labour. - Proverbs 21: 25

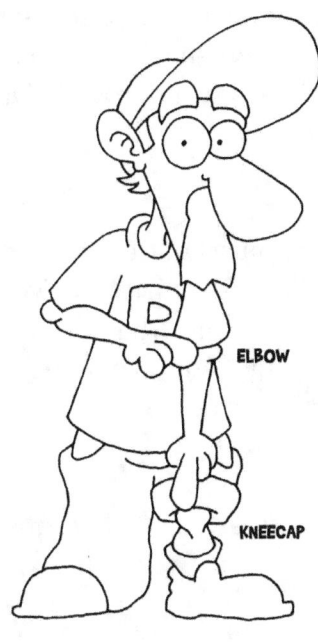
ELBOW

KNEECAP

Being lazy leads to poverty and causes many health problems. The body was designed to move. That's why we were made with elbows, ankles and knee caps. These are like hinges for our body's moving parts. We are supposed to move. Think about it.

Normal natural exercise consists of walking, running, reaching, bending and lifting. It's how we were designed. There are healthy benefits from exercising. It help us to feel better, have more energy and possibly live longer.

Here are six benefits that I found from the Internet:

Exercise controls weight
Exercise can help prevent excess weight gain or help maintain weight loss. Physical activity helps you burn calories. The more intense the activity, the more calories you burn.

Exercise fights against health problems
Exercise keeps your blood flowing smoothly and decreases your risk of cardiovascular diseases. As a matter of fact, regular physical activity can help you prevent or manage a wide range of health problems and concerns, including stroke, metabolic syndrome, type 2 diabetes, depression, certain types of cancer and arthritis.

Exercise improves mood
Physical activity stimulates various brain chemicals that may

leave you feeling happier and more relaxed. You may also feel better about your appearance and yourself when you exercise regularly, which can boost your confidence and improve your self-esteem.

Exercise boosts energy
Regular physical activity can improve your muscle strength and boost your endurance. Exercise and physical activity deliver oxygen and nutrients to your tissues and help your cardiovascular system work more efficiently. And when your heart and lungs work more efficiently, you have more energy.

Exercise promotes better sleep
Regular physical activity can help you fall asleep faster and deepen your sleep.

Exercise can be fun
Exercise and physical activity can be a fun way to spend some time. It gives you a chance to unwind, enjoy the outdoors or simply engage in activities that make you happy. Physical activity can also help you connect with family or friends in a fun social setting.

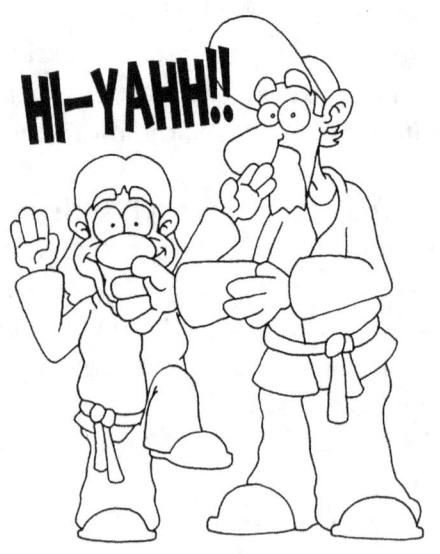

Exercise can be accomplished through normal everyday activities. You don't necessarily have to go to the gym to do it. You can walk up and down steps, walk to your mailbox, lift items in your home and create physical activities to do with your family like a game of horseshoes outside. The trick is to simply move body parts. It really doesn't matter what you do. Get everybody involved. Grab your spouse and do some playful Kung Fu fighting in the living room. Just make it fun.

Food In The Bible

There are many foods mentioned in the Bible. I found this interesting and thought I should share it with you. Many of these are foods that we eat today. Check it out!

Seasonings, Spices and Herbs
Anise (Matthew 23:23 KJV)
Coriander (Exodus 16:31; Numbers 11:7)
Cinnamon (Exodus 30:23; Revelation 18:13)
Cumin (Isaiah 28:25; Matthew 23:23)
Dill (Matthew 23:23)
Garlic (Numbers 11:5)
Mint (Matthew 23:23; Luke 11:42)
Mustard (Matthew 13:31)
Rue (Luke 11:42)
Salt (Ezra 6:9; Job 6:6)

Fruits and Nuts
Apples (Song of Solomon 2:5)
Almonds (Genesis 43:11; Numbers 17:8)
Dates (2 Samuel 6:19; 1 Chronicles 16:3)
Figs (Nehemiah 13:15; Jeremiah 24:1-3)
Grapes (Leviticus 19:10; Deuteronomy 23:24)
Melons (Numbers 11:5; Isaiah 1:8)
Olives (Isaiah 17:6; Micah 6:15)
Pistachio Nuts (Genesis 43:11)

Pomegranates (Numbers 20:5; Deuteronomy 8:8)
Raisins (Numbers 6:3; 2 Samuel 6:19)
Sycamore Fruit (Psalm 78:47; Amos 7:14)

Vegetables and Legumes .
Beans (2 Samuel 17:28; Ezekiel 4:9)
Cucumbers (Numbers 11:5)
Gourds (2 Kings 4:39)
Leeks (Numbers 11:5)
Lentils (Genesis 25:34; 2 Samuel 17:28; Ezekiel 4:9)
Onions (Numbers 11:5)

Grains
Barley (Deuteronomy 8:8; Ezekiel 4:9)
Bread (Genesis 25:34; 2 Samuel 6:19; 16:1; Mark 8:14)
Corn (Matthew 12:1; KJV - refers to "grain" such as wheat or barley)
Flour (2 Samuel 17:28; 1 Kings 17:12)
Millet (Ezekiel 4:9)
Spelt (Ezekiel 4:9)
Unleavened Bread (Genesis 19:3; Exodus 12:20)
Wheat (Ezra 6:9; Deuteronomy 8:8)

Fish
Matthew 15:36
John 21:11-13

Fowl
Partridge (1 Samuel 26:20; Jeremiah 17:11)
Pigeon (Genesis 15:9; Leviticus 12:8)
Quail (Psalm 105:40)
Dove (Leviticus 12:8)

Animal Meats
Calf (Proverbs 15:17; Luke 15:23)
Goat (Genesis 27:9)
Lamb (2 Samuel 12:4)
Oxen (1 Kings 19:21)
Sheep (Deuteronomy 14:4)
Venison (Genesis 27:7 KJV)

Dairy
Butter (Proverbs 30:33)
Cheese (2 Samuel 17:29; Job 10:10)
Curds (Isaiah 7:15)
Milk (Exodus 33:3; Job 10:10; Judges 5:25)

Miscellaneous
Eggs (Job 6:6; Luke 11:12)
Grape Juice (Numbers 6:3)
Honey (Exodus 33:3; Deuteronomy 8:8; Judges 14:8-9)
Locust (Mark 1:6)
Olive Oil (Ezra 6:9; Deuteronomy 8:8)
Vinegar (Ruth 2:14; John 19:29)
Wine (Ezra 6:9; John 2:1-10)

The Daniel Diet

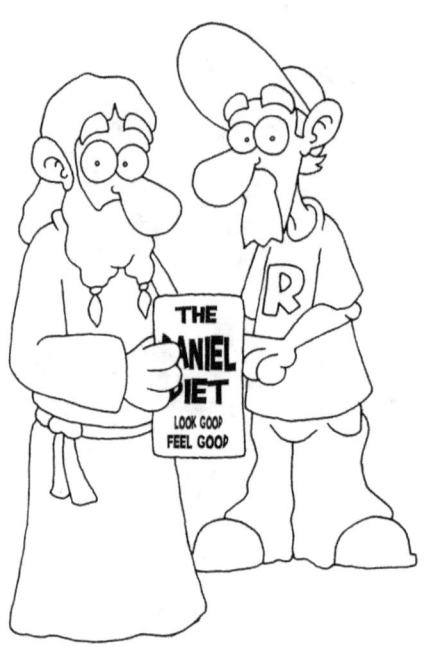

But Daniel purposed in his heart that he would not defile himself with the portion of the king's meat, nor with the wine which he drank: therefore he requested of the prince of the eunuchs that he might not defile himself. Now God had brought Daniel into favour and tender love with the prince of the eunuchs. And the prince of the eunuchs said unto Daniel, I fear my lord the king, who hath appointed your meat and your drink: for why should he see your faces worse liking than the children which are of your sort? then shall ye make me endanger my head to the king. Then said Daniel to Melzar, whom the prince of the eunuchs had set over Daniel, Hananiah, Mishael, and Azariah, Prove thy servants, I beseech thee, ten days; and let them give us pulse to eat, and water to drink. Then let our countenances be looked upon before thee, and the countenance of the children that eat of the portion of the king's meat: and as thou seest, deal with thy servants. So he consented to them in this matter, and proved them ten days. And at the end of ten days their countenances appeared fairer and fatter in flesh than all the children which did eat the portion of the king's meat. - Daniel 1: 8-14

In those days I Daniel was mourning three full weeks. I ate no pleasant bread, neither came flesh nor wine in my mouth, neither did I anoint myself at all, till three whole weeks were fulfilled. - Daniel 10: 2, 3

Some people practice the Daniel Diet for their health. There are two types. There is the 10-day Daniel Diet which consists of eating vegetables and drinking water only. There's also the 21-day diet which includes eating whole grains, beans, fruits, seeds and drinking liquids such as all-natural fruit juices.

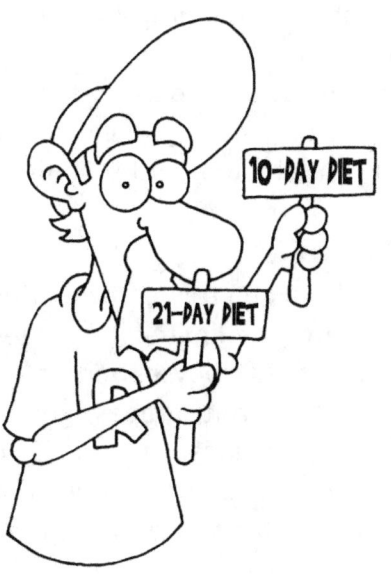

The Daniel Diet isn't something new. People do it to help themselves spiritually and make their bodies feel better. The idea behind it is found in the Bible in the Book of Daniel.

Daniel 1: 8-14
Daniel and three of his buddies were taken captive by the Babylonian army when Judah was seized. They were chosen to serve in the king's palace and were required to eat a diet that went against their tradition. Daniel asked if they could be allowed to abstain from the 'king's meat' for 10 days. He allowed it and the results were positive.

Daniel 10: 2, 3
This was a fast that Daniel did to spiritually connect to God. He did this for three whole weeks.

The Daniel Diet is not a diet designed for weight loss, but is rather meant as a physical experience that reflects a spiritual commitment leading to deeper insights from God. If you're a Christian, you will cleanse your body, mind and spirit with the Daniel Diet when you use it as a method of sacrifice unto God, combined with prayer and daily Bible reading.

If you are considering doing the Daniel Diet, remember to eat foods that are sugar and chemical free. Here are foods to include in your diet during the Daniel Diet:

All Fruits
These can be fresh, frozen, dried, juiced or canned. Fruits include but are not limited to apples, apricots, bananas, blackberries, blueberries, boysenberries, cantaloupe, cherries, cranberries, figs, grapefruit, grapes, guava, honeydew melon, kiwi, lemons, limes, mangoes, nectarines, oranges, papayas, peaches, pears, pineapples, plums, prunes, raisins, raspberries, strawberries, tangelos, tangerines and watermelon.

All Vegetables
These can be fresh, frozen, dried, juiced or canned. Vegetables include but are not limited to artichokes, asparagus, beets, broccoli, Brussels sprouts, cabbage, carrots, cauliflower, celery, chili peppers, collard greens, corn, cucumbers, eggplant, garlic, ginger root, kale, leeks, lettuce, mushrooms, mustard greens, okra, onions, parsley, potatoes, radishes, rutabagas, scallions, spinach, sprouts, squashes, sweet potatoes, tomatoes, turnips, watercress, yams and zucchini. Veggie burgers are an option if you are not allergic to soy.

All Whole Grains
These include but are not limited to whole wheat, brown rice, millet, quinoa, oats, barley, grits, whole wheat pasta, whole

wheat tortillas, rice cakes and popcorn.

All Nuts And Seeds
These include but are not limited to sunflower seeds, cashews, peanuts and sesame. Also nut butters including peanut butter.

All Legumes
These can be canned or dried. Legumes include but are not limited to dried beans, pinto beans, split peas, lentils, black eyed peas, kidney beans, black beans, cannellini beans and white beans.

All Quality Oils
These include but are not limited to olive, canola, grape seed, peanut, and sesame.

Beverages
These can be spring water, distilled water or other pure waters.

Other Foods
These can be tofu, soy products, vinegar, seasonings, salt, herbs and spices.

Foods To Avoid On The Daniel Diet
- All meat and animal products including but not limited to beef, lamb, pork, poultry, and fish.
- All dairy products including but not limited to milk, cheese, cream, butter, and eggs.
- All sweeteners including but not limited to sugar, raw sugar, honey, syrups, molasses, and cane juice.
- All leavened bread including Ezekiel Bread (it contains yeast and honey) and baked goods.
- All refined and processed food products including but not

limited to artificial flavorings, food additives, chemicals, white rice, white flour and foods that contain artificial preservatives.

- All deep fried foods including but not limited to potato chips, French fries and corn chips.
- All solid fats including shortening, margarine, lard and foods high in fat.
- Beverages including but not limited to coffee, tea, herbal teas, carbonated beverages, energy drinks and alcohol.

The Daniel Diet mentioned in the Bible from Chapter 10 is very similar to how life is today. We basically eat what the higher authorities provide for us at our grocery stores. It could be considered the 'king's meat'. Maybe breaking away from the worldly system and choosing our own foods would be to our advantage. Let's try it for 10 days. What could it hurt?

Putting The Pieces Together

The great thing about life is that, if we ever get lost along the way, we can always turn around and ask for help.

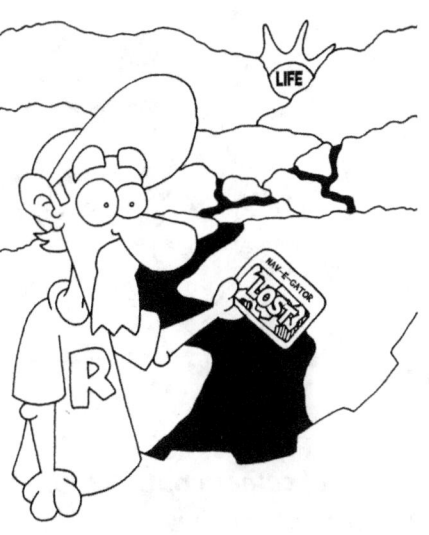

Spiritually, if you're tired of the destructive direction your life is heading, we can always look up and ask for God to step in and lead the way. If you're not saved, you can pray and ask Him to save you. By doing so, He can help you put your life into perspective and direct you on a better path.

When it comes to our health, if we begin seeing signs that our bodies show us about the unhealthy way we are living, we can stop, look for help and make the proper adjustments.

God and the Bible are always there to help us get on track. Prayer is our best tool to connect with the One that created us. He knows our bodies and what it will take to help us become healthier and live better. We are His creation. He holds all of the answers. We should speak to Him, give Him our worries and allow Him to help us through them.

The Bible was written by God through man. When it comes to health and spiritual matters, we should use it as a guide. Apply it to our life and do what it says. It can only make us better.

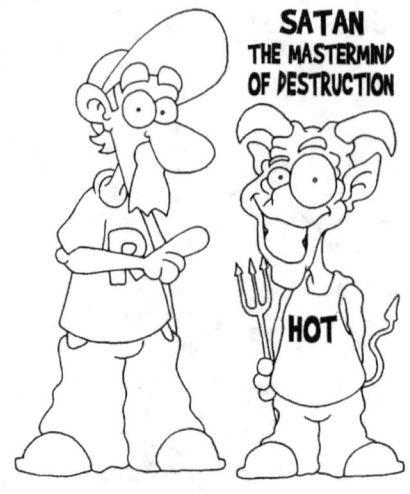

SATAN THE MASTERMIND OF DESTRUCTION

Yes, the world is a mess. Everyone has some kind of problem, whether it be our health, finances or relationships and that's just naming a few. But, remember, there is a mastermind behind all of this destruction. His name is Satan. I'm sure you've heard of him? He is actively participating in the affairs of the world today with the purpose of doing some damage. You are one of his targets, too.

The thief cometh not, but for to steal, and to kill, and to destroy: I am come that they might have life, and that they might have it more abundantly. - John 10: 10

God should be the One we turn to with all of our problems. He can help. He gives life and wants us all to enjoy it. All we have to do is reach out to Him.

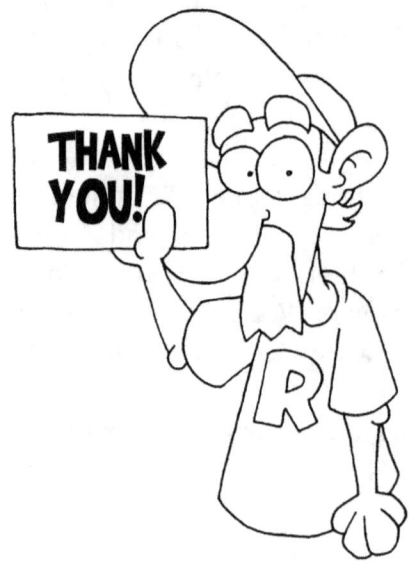

I would like to thank you for reading this guide today. I hope you received something from it. I know I did. I believe this is our wake-up call to learn more about the foods we put into our bodies. We need to get up from our comfort zones and do something that will benefit our health.

Let's live and let God lead the way! Ya know?

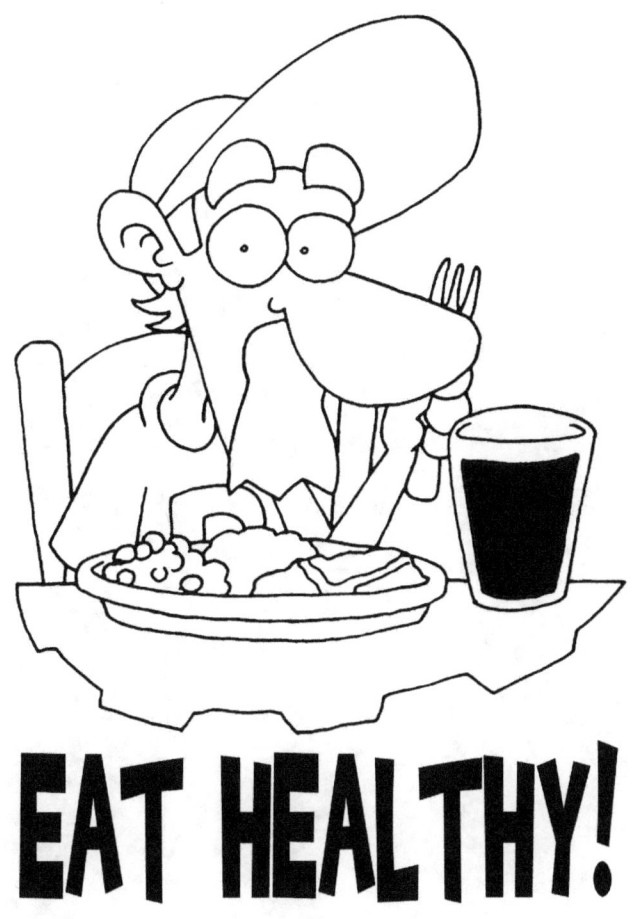

About The
Author/Cartoonist

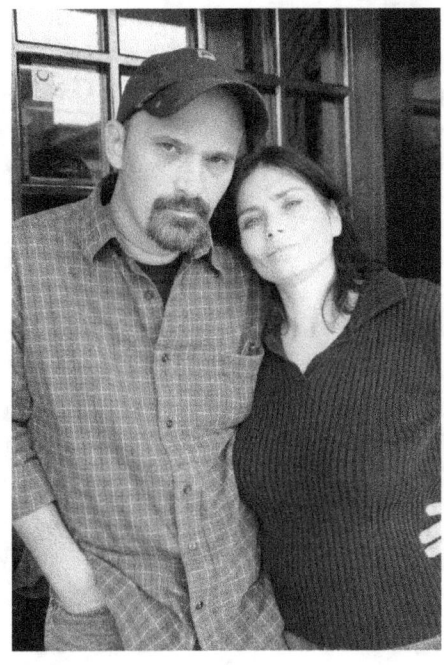

This is the section of a book where an author tells the world of all his or her accomplishments in life. They usually list their qualifications, certifications, doctrinations, and give their explanations of why they think they are such a cool author. But that's not going to happen today.

You see, Jeff Todd is just a simple man with a simple name and lives in a simple part of the world where the only people that know him are some of the ones he went to school with and his family and close friends. That's it!

Jeff was born in Newnan, Georgia in 1969. If you did the math, you would probably realize he was older than dirt. He and his wife, Frances have been married since 1989 and are doing their best to raise their four children, just like every honest American does. One of the best things they have ever done as a family was allow the Lord to lead, guide, and direct them.

At the age of 14, Jeff asked Jesus to come into his life and save him. Ever since then, his Christian life has been a learning experience. The lessons he has learned were on-hand experiences that you may not find in reading inspirational books. Twenty four years later, this turned into a ministry to help others know more about being a Christian and how to grow, encouraging others to step out of their boat and become what the Lord wants them to be, and most importantly to reach out to the lost that don't know Jesus as their Savior and lead them to Him. It doesn't take a genius to do this! Actually it's so simple that even a Redneck can do it!

Jeff uses his God-given talents, gifts, and skills to do what the Lord has called him to do. It's not much, but undoubtedly God is able to use him anyway. He is just the vessel. Music, writing, drawing, and a loud mouth are the main tools he is using for the Lord currently and he loves it! Jeff hopes you get the spiritual help you need from it.

About The
Ministry

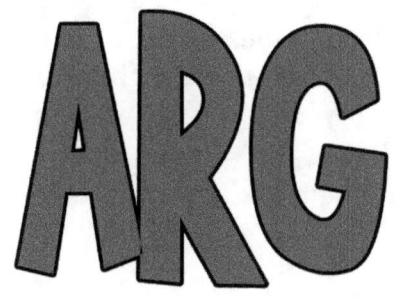

A Redneck's Guide Series began as blogs back in 2007 and has now turned into a series of books. That's pretty exciting for a redneck writer/cartoonist living in Small Town, Georgia. Ain't it?

But, what's it all for? Why A Redneck's Guide? Good question.

As you already know, the Bible is our source of information; our spiritual nourishment to help us grow as Christians. However, it seems that many of us are guilty of not reading it. We rely on our preachers and teachers to do it for us. The sad thing is that, in a world of false teaching (which is warned about in the Bible), we may be receiving some bad information and accepting it as truth. But, you know, this could easily be resolved by reading the Bible for ourselves.

Recently, I did some research on the internet and discovered that some of the main reasons people don't read the Bible is because they are either too lazy or that they don't understand it. That's interesting.

It was laid on my heart back in 2007 to step out of my comfort zone and share God's Word with people. I felt the 'calling' to use my God-given talents and to put the Bible out there to help folks understand what it's saying. Pushing aside any religious denomination, I went at this with an open mind and read these books of the Bible for myself and allowed it to speak to me personally. I would then take this information and write about it in my own simple-minded words. I'm a Redneck – what would you expect? Now, the cartoons I draw for it are an added bonus to help the reader visually in receiving the message. Plus, they're kinda cool to look at. I personally like to read books with pictures. How about you?

This is my 'calling' – a Christian Redneck writer/cartoonist. Sounds funny, don't it?

Go ye therefore, and teach all nations, baptizing them in the name of the Father, and of the Son, and of the Holy Ghost: Teaching them to observe all things whatsoever I have commanded you: and, lo, I am with you alway, even unto the end of the world. Amen. - Matthew 28: 19, 20

Even though the books from A Redneck's Guide look funny or weird, they're very serious. There are currently 34 books in the series and they belong to the Lord. He's in charge and I'm just a simple servant.

Just know that A Redneck's Guide Series is about sharing God's Word with people in a simple and easy-to-understand way. That's the way it should be.

Always keep this ministry in your prayers and continue telling others about it.

God bless ya'll!

More From

A Redneck's Guide Series

To Being A Christian
- The Simple-Minded Folk Edition
- Prison Ministry Edition
- Street Ministry Edition
- Toon-Up Edition
- French Edition
- Spanish Edition
- Kindle Edition
- Audiobook
- Audiobook on CD
- Comic Book Edition

The Gospel Series
- Behind The Miracles
- To The Pair-O-Bulls
- The Redneck School Of Rock
- Jesus – Outside The Box
- The Gospel – Kindle Edition in 8 Different Languages

For The Kids
- Getcha Doodlin' On! - Activity Book

The 5-Minute Sermons
- Volume 1
- Volume 2
- Volume 3

- Volume 4

The Church Letters
- Galatians
- Ephesians
- Philippians
- Thessalonians
- Corinthians
- Colossians
- To The Church Letters - Kindle Edition

The New Testament
- Row Man! Row!
- The Axe Of The Apostles
- Dear John
- The Ultimate Rock Band 5
- Revelation - The Duct Tape Removed
- He Brews!
- Row Man! Row! - Kindle Edition
- The Axe Of The Apostles - Kindle Edition
- Dear John - Kindle Edition
- The Ultimate Rock Band 5 - Kindle Edition
- Revelation - The Duct Tape Removed - Kindle Edition
- He Brews! - Kindle Edition

The Spiritual Duct Tape Series
- To Stayin' Married
- To Being A Dad
- To Eatin' Right!
- To Stayin' Married – Kindle Edition
- To Being A Dad – Kindle Edition
- To Eatin' Right! – Kindle Edition

Miscellaneous Books/CDs
- A Modern Day Psalm
- A Work Through Me
- New Testament: A Simple Man's Commentary – Volume 1
- New Testament: A Simple Man's Commentary – Volume 2
- A Work Through Me (Kindle)
- NT: A Simple Man's Commentary – Volume 1 (Kindle)
- NT: A Simple Man's Commentary – Volume 2 (Kindle)
- Work Through Me – Audio CD

Visit us at:
www.ARGseries.com
www.ARGstuff.com
www.ToonItUpGraphics.com
Or find us on Facebook

www.ingramcontent.com/pod-product-compliance
Lightning Source LLC
Chambersburg PA
CBHW062014280526
45787CB00005B/2096